Age Smart Fitness

All I Really Need Is My Health

Practical & Inspirational Guide For a Healthier, Happier You

MOVE, LIVE & FEEL GREAT

Lisa McLellan

Age Smart Fitness

All I Really Need Is My Health

Published by Age Smart Fitness
ISBN-13: 978-0-9949512-0-5
ISBN-10: 0994951205

Book Website
www.agesmartfitness.com
Email: agesmartfitness@gmail.com

Give comment on the book at:
www.agesmartfitness.com/book

Printed in U.S.A

TABLE OF CONTENTS

INTRODUCTION

Over the last nine years I have been observing something most remarkable, something which keeps me very excited and motivated about my work, something which moves me to continually develop my ideas and abilities. That something is my clients and their transformations. I would like to dedicate this book to their many successes and applaud the efforts they have made to improve their health and live their best lives.

Before I continue, I would like to underline the single most important factor that will have an impact on your fitness and well-being: CONSTANCY. Constancy will be the key to your success. Constancy yields results. Results keep you motivated. Baby steps involve smaller more manageable efforts. Baby steps over time produce big changes in both body and mind. And that is what I am proposing to do with you in this book. So get ready for a profound and meaningful life change.

Since 2006 I have been writing a monthly 50+ Fit Tip for the Main-Street newspaper. To date, I have written over 100 tips. This book is based on a collection of those tips. Over the next 12 months I will give you one easy, doable lifestyle habit to practise every month. We will build on these habits, month by month, layering healthy lifestyle habits into our daily routines. You will be surprised and enchanted by how a few simple changes in your everyday life can have an enduring and profound impact on your health and happiness. Each month will contain 4 tips; one per week. Week 1 will lay out the challenge of the month and explain its benefits. Weeks 2 and 3 will offer related tips to educate, motivate and inspire you further. Week 4 will consist of an anecdote, a personal story, something meaningful in my life that I want to share.

The book is divided into three parts:

> Part One: **Laying The Foundations**
> Part Two: **The Inward Journey**
> Part Three: **Spreading Your Wings**

Each part offers a different kind of challenge and encourages a different level of integration. I hope you will enjoy the journey. I certainly have.

Now, here are some of the outstanding accomplishments achieved by my clients as a result of my Age Smart Fitness program.

Jacques, at 79, survived an adverse reaction to a surgical intervention, which would have killed him had he not been in such good physical shape. We worked together twice a week. Ginette, 55, put her passion behind getting into shape and lost 61 pounds in one year, completely transforming herself. She even quit smoking. She takes five classes a week. Kay, 70+, has improved her posture and is now a half inch taller. Her doctor couldn't believe it and measured her twice! She has been taking one class a week since September. Cristina, 60+ has overcome annoying back pain and looks fantastic in her new connected, firm, trim body. Cristina takes four classes a week. Jean, 60+, is more supple since he started Yoga. He feels so much better too. He takes two Yoga classes a week. Nicole who takes five classes a week, lost 10 pounds in three weeks and feels like a champion. In the Gym, in stretch class and with the help of specialists Anne has worked with great diligence, overcoming injuries from a serious accident. This year's results are even better than last. Cumulative results can move mountains.

Barb is enjoying more flexibility and less pain. Her husband is working steadily as well to get back into tip-top shape after heart surgery. Richard has been hard at work since September and as a result has lost weight, improved his heart health and upped his muscular strength. He's also wearing a big smile. Mary has patiently overcome back trouble and is on her way to dancing up a storm. Eleanor has transformed herself into a light and elegant being. Marguerite just keeps on ticking and ticking and she is … I'm not allowed to say but I'm impressed! Agnes likes a challenge. She keeps her muscles in really good shape that's why she only looks just over 60! Claude has overcome debilitating neck and upper-back pain by taking one Stretch and Strengthen class a week and doing my 15-minute Chair Program DVD every morning. Lise has lost 30 pounds in six months and feels better than ever. Her success is supported by both exercise and visits to the naturopath.

I don't want to forget those who have reduced or eliminated their prescribed medications, those who have found solace and strength after difficult challenges such as injuries, surgeries and illness or death of a spouse or parent. I can think of many more examples but am running out of space. So, bravo to all my clients for their efforts, their constancy and their progress! Five gold stars.

I encourage each and every one of you to take an active role in your health and well-being so you too can benefit from some of the amazing results which await you. I am here to guide and motivate you ... with my big black boots (to kick your butt) and my velvet gloves (for the sensitive you). Stay active, be constant and watch the gold stars pile up around you. Twinkle. Twinkle. Twinkle.

I want to share with you now the top 5 regrets from palliative care nurse Bronnie Ware's book, *The Top Five Regrets of the Dying: A Life Transformed by the Dearly Departing*. Let us not fall victim to these regrets when we still have time to act.

1. **I wish I'd had the courage to live a life true to myself, not the life others expected of me.** "Most people had not honoured even a half of their dreams and had to die knowing that it was due to choices they had made, or not made. Health brings a freedom very few realize, until they no longer have it."

2. **I wish I hadn't worked so hard.**
   "All of the men I nursed deeply regretted spending so much of their lives on the treadmill of a work existence. They missed their children's youth and their partner's companionship."

3. **I wish I'd had the courage to express my feelings.**
   "Many people suppressed their feelings in order to keep peace with others. As a result, they settled for a mediocre existence and never became who they were truly capable of becoming. Many developed illnesses relating to the bitterness and resentment they carried as a result."

4. **I wish I had stayed in touch with my friends.**
   "There were many deep regrets about not giving friendships the time and effort that they deserved. Everyone misses their friends when they are dying."

5. **I wish that I had let myself be happier.**
   "Many did not realize until the end that happiness is a choice. They had stayed stuck in old patterns and habits. The so-called "comfort" of familiarity overflowed into their emotions, as well as their physical lives. Fear of change had them pretending to others, and to their selves, that they were content, when deep within, they longed to laugh properly and have silliness in their life again."

I am making a promise to you. So here it goes. If you practise the 12 lifestyle habits that I have chosen for you over the next year, you will be equipped to address each one of these regrets. You will come to live a better, more radiant life. If you would like to have me coach you through the process to help you succeed, you can join my on-line coaching community at www.agesmartfitness.com. As part of this coaching you will receive the Fit Tip of the week in your inbox, along with a coaching video of me and my guests to keep you motivated and on track, as well as a workbook in which to record your progress. You can post questions, share and exchange in our private Facebook group for extra support and encouragement. Let's do this together, you and I, and transform our lives in unimaginable ways for the better.

Move, Live and Feel Great.

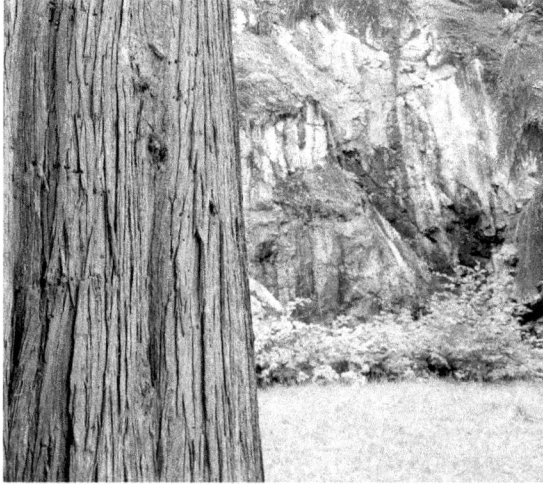

PART ONE
LAYING THE FOUNDATIONS

"Aging is real. Your body does change.
But your body and mind are equal to
what you do to maintain it".

Dr. Doug Clement

INVITATION
A FRESH START

This could be a new beginning, if you decide. What will you choose? What does your heart desire?

Please allow me to remind you:
1. You and only you can be responsible for yourself, your health and your well being. That goes for men too. Lol
2. What you think and believe will make a difference in the life you create for yourself.
3. What you choose to do or not do will have a profound impact on the quality of your life and its outcome.
4. What you eat and drink will determine in large part the state of your health.
5. Your commitment to physical activity will be reflected in the level of health and fitness you achieve.

You will either build energy or lose energy depending on your choices and actions. Where does discipline come from? Will? Motivation? Energy? There are many answers to these questions and we will get to that. But without doubt, the first step to finding the answers comes from choosing to care for yourself and commiting totally to that choice.

Remember that in caring for yourself, you are also showing your love for those who care about you.

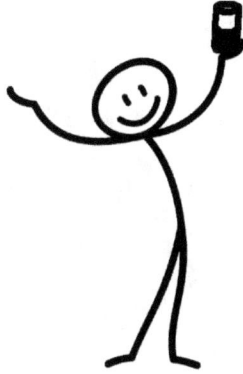

MONTH ONE
Challenge of the Month: HYDRATE

> Drink 1 cup of warm water mixed with the juice of
> half a lemon first thing every morning

If for some reason you can't tolerate the lemon juice you can:
1. Dilute with more water
2. Replace the lemon with 1 tablespoon of organic apple cider vinegar
3. Use the lemon juice and organic lemon rind in your salad dressing, on vegetables, fish, etc.
4. Use an alkaline water filter - I recommend Vitev. http://vitev.refr.cc/2D3BJF8

WEEK 1
WATER AND LEMON MAGIC

The way you start each day is incredibly important. What you do first thing in the morning matters. When you start the day off right, it's easier for you to make good choices for yourself the rest of the day. Although your mind might try to convince you that you have to check emails, take the dog out, that you can't be late for work or that you don't have time it simply isn't true!

Challenge One: Drink one cup of warm water mixed with the juice of half a lemon first thing every morning.

Here are a few reasons why drinking one cup of warm water mixed with the juice of half a lemon every morning is a good choice. It is also an easy choice, which means you can do it.

1. **Boosts the immune system:** Lemons are high in Vitamin C and potassium. Vitamin C is great for fighting colds, and potassium stimulates brain and nerve function and helps control blood pressure.
2. **Balances pH:** Lemons are incredibly alkaline. While they are acidic on their own, inside our bodies they're alkaline. An alkaline body is key to good health.
3. **Helps with weight loss:** Lemons are high in pectin fibre, and this helps fight hunger cravings. It also has been shown that people who maintain a more alkaline pH lose weight faster.
4. **Helps keep the skin clear:** Vitamin C helps diminish wrinkles and clear up blemishes. Lemon water purges toxins from the blood which helps keep the skin clear as well.
5. **Aids digestion:** The warm water serves to stimulate our gastrointestinal tract and peristalsis—the wave of muscle contractions within the intestinal walls that keeps things moving. Lemons and limes are also high in minerals and vitamins and help loosen toxins in the digestive tract.
6. **Hydrates the lymph system:** Water is the essence of life. It is the most important nutrient in our bodies, making up roughly 70 percent of our muscle and brain tissue. Only oxygen is craved by the body more than water. Start every day with

water to help prevent dehydration. When your body is dehydrated it can't function properly. This leads to toxic buildup, stress, constipation, headaches, fatigue, bloating, problems concentrating, drowsiness, dry skin and lips, cold hands and feet, impatience and irritability. Your adrenal glands secrete a hormone that regulates water levels and the concentration of minerals, such as sodium, in your body, helping you to stay hydrated. Chronic dehydration, from which most of us suffer, leads to adrenal fatigue thereby affecting the performance of the adrenal glands.

So go ahead and drink a cup of warm water mixed with the juice of half a lemon first thing every morning. Observe how you feel as the month progresses. An important part of integrating healthy lifestyle habits and making them stick is to become aware of the impact that the new habit has on the way you feel. So drop all of your excuses and do this with me for one month. Watch how one simple little change can make you feel better!

WEEK 2
THE PROBLEM OF PAIN

Arrgh pain! Many of my clients suffer from it; perhaps you do to. Headache pain, shoulder pain, elbow pain, back pain, leg pain, knee pain, foot pain, *pain in the neck* pain. More often than not we simply try to ignore pain in the hopes that it will go away. Sometimes it does, sometimes it doesn't. Pain is a sign from your body that something is amiss and needs attending to. Therefore, the sooner you address pain and take care of yourself, the better. Pain affects how you feel, and interferes with what you can or can't do. Left untreated the problem can worsen, creating more pain and a more serious problem that still needs to be dealt with! Pain comes in varying degrees of seriousness: aches and pains, pain stemming from old or new injuries and chronic pain related to disease and/or other factors, as well as combinations thereof.

Aches and Pains
Aches and pains, that are not as a result of chronic diseases such as arthritis, osteoarthritis and fibromyalgia for example, can most certainly be eliminated. This type of pain generally stems from bad posture, incorrect biomechanics, poor food choices and stress. Stress on the body causes body/mind tension that affects all aspects of the physical body. Bad posture affects muscular tone and balance, skeletal alignment and breathing. Proper skeletal alignment provides structural support to the body and is necessary for efficient biomechanics (the way we move our bodies) and healthy joints. When we accumulate muscular tension in specific areas (neck, shoulders, back) these areas become stiff and painful. Over time the muscles shorten and lose their natural flexibility as a result of habitual contraction. Muscles are designed to both contract and lengthen. When this natural action is restricted, range of motion is decreased. Decreased range of motion limits mobility, and muscles become weak from lack of use. The fascia and connective tissue become rigid and constricted. As the body becomes more and more bound by rigidity, bad posture and restricted range of motion, the natural equilibrium and harmony of the body are adversely affected. The resulting imbalance causes wear and tear on the joints, ligaments and tendons as well as chronic stress in the corresponding myofascial structures causing for example, back pain and headaches. Does this sound like you?

Pain creates fear of pain. Fear of pain creates tension and compensation - to try and avoid the pain. Tension and compensation create greater imbalance, new pain and on and on it goes. Aging and the force of unconscious habits compound the problem. As does gravity. In good posture, gravity acts to keep you up straight. In bad posture, gravity causes you to shrink and curve down. Oh lalalala! Don't we know it? When clients first come to me many appear to be prisoners of their own bodies. This may sound a little harsh but it was this observation that motivated me to find solutions for clients suffering from the aches and pain of aging and develop the Age Smart Fitness program for which I am so appreciated.

Chronic Pain

I want to acknowledge those of you who suffer from chronic pain and share my compassion for your pain and trials. Sadly, I do not have any magic cure to offer you. I asked my Dad, who suffers from arthritis and asthma, what he does to deal with the pain and he replied, in a most sincere way, "You learn to live with it." That is the essence of pain management. Pain management, like all other health matters, brings us back to square one: mental discipline, nutrition, exercise and the guidance of healthcare professionals.

I understand that it is difficult to feel good when you feel bad. But what can you do? In the end each one of us will have to find our own way to manage pain. So here goes, my practical tips for dealing with chronic pain.

1. **Mind over matter.** Eliminate the stressors in your life. This is a must. Learn to calm your mind and be positive. Redirect your attention away from pain by thinking of something else, by staying busy and interested. Over time, as you learn to shift your attention, you will become less governed by pain. Take a class in relaxation or mindfulness practice. Find a hobby.

2. **You are what you eat.** Address your eating habits. Do not underestimate the importance of diet. Chronic diseases are very affected by what we eat and can be aggravated by inappropriate food choices or, conversely improved by a wholesome diet. Supplementation, although a controversial subject, provides relief from pain for many people. Consult a specialist.

3. **Regular gentle exercise.** Reduce the range of motion, reduce the intensity, refrain from movements which cause pain or ag-

gravate the problem. Shorten your bouts of exercise or physical activity but continue to engage in such activity regularly. Swimming is great because the body does not bear weight on the joints. Gentle, conscious stretching is excellent for eliminating stiffness/pain and is recommended as a daily exercise for arthritis. Body/mind disciplines such as Qigong, Tai Chi or gentle Yoga are all-around positive. Walk if you can. For osteoarthritis, do strength training (with proper technique). Preserve your joints by honouring your limits. Do not overdo it. The "no pain, no gain" motto is not for you. Although it is vexing (to put it mildly) to lose some of our past freedoms, let us not forget to enjoy the beauty and pleasure life is offering right now.

4. **Attention to medication.** A change in prescription dosage, type or brand may produce very surprising results. Consult your doctor. Regular exercise can help reduce your need for medication. For other options consult a specialist in alternative medicine.

Pain requires tender loving care, patience and perseverance. You simply can't force pain or injury away. Taking pills is a solution (sometimes a necessary solution) but pills do not necessarily cure pain. Participating actively in your health and well-being will ultimately be the key to your success. Maintaining a healthy lifestyle daily will guarantee it.

Post Rehabilitation

Post rehab starts once the doctor has sent you home and your physiotherapy has been completed. It is the transition period. You are on your own but not really up and running. You are in a weakened state, not yet fully mended still fragile. Truth be told, your muscles have lost their strength and tone. Your range of motion is reduced and movements may still be painful. Your endurance (except maybe for pain) is down. Even going for a walk can be hard. You are more easily winded and lack energy. Your vitality is low - a result of the healing process or the side effects of medication. You may even be a little depressed or irritable … even though you are trying your best to put on a good face. You may be feeling all or some of these things. Some days may be good, some not. You may experience an emotional and physical roller coaster ride, especially if the healing process is long and slow.

Well guess what? You are normal! You are in a de-conditioned state. No matter how good you are feeling, don't forget that. You are healing; rebuilding your tissues and your fitness reserve. You are contending with recovery combined with the reality of aging (refer to Month 3, week 3 - The Physiology of Aging). You can improve this state of being only by actively working on it. I invite you to be mindful of the steps in the healing process and to respect them. What you do or choose to not do during this period, will determine the success of your rehabilitation and your return to fitness and vitality. Please do not underestimate the importance of the post-rehab phase of your healing process. Do not neglect it.

The two bigest mistakes made during the post-rehab phase are:

1. **Doing too much, too fast.** Be patient; re-injuring yourself sets you further back than where you were when you started. Don't make that mistake please!

2. **Not doing anything.** Be proactive and get moving gently. Don't be fearful. Take responsibility for your healing so you can once again fully embrace life.

I send out my blessings and positive good vibrations to my Dad, my friend Hans and anyone else who is in a healing process. Listen to your body. Be smart. Be disciplined. Do the exercises the physio gave you to do. Stay positive. Enjoy the process and learn about yourself. I'll be thinking about you and those who are helping and supporting you. Big hug.

WEEK 3
THE GIFT OF WATER

Drink water. Drink water to cure asthma, allergies, dyspepsia (digestive disorders), rheumatoid arthritis, angina, hypertension, low back pain, leg pain in walking, excess body weight, migraines and constipation. Drink water as prevention against the onset of chronic degenerative disease. Drink water to prevent premature aging. That is what F. Batmanghelidj, MD, advises in his book *Your Body's Many Cries for Water.* www.watercure.com

He demonstrates, through an in-depth physiological study of the human body, that chronic dehydration (lack of water) is the root cause of most major degenerative diseases. His solution: drink adequate amounts of water daily to meet the body's needs. He points out that the natural solution of drinking water is not of interest to mainstream medicine because it is not a money-making proposition for the "business" of health care. Imagine treating patients with water rather than pills! Revolutionary! He argues that dehydration has to be ruled out before prescribing medications such as antacids, anti-inflammatory drugs, pain medications or anti-depressants for emerging disease symptoms. The reason for this is that medications silence the body's signals of thirst and more importantly, they do not address the cause.

He has proven that drinking water is a cure for many degenerative diseases that are considered incurable, especially if put into practice before irreparable damage to the cells, organs and joints has occurred as a result of dehydration. This is a radical point of view and very well defended in his book. Even though Dr. Batmanghelidj is not a gifted writer, I recommend that you read his book. The facts are equally fascinating and troublesome in their implications. The good news: the solution is readily available in your kitchens and you can immediately start to address those troublesome conditions and improve your health!

Most doctors would roll their eyes and think "quack". I know my father who is a doctor would. He does not believe that water is important in the healing of disease. Dr. Batmanghelidj mentions that doctors have this attitude towards water because the medical paradigm upon which their training is based focuses on the 25 percent of solids that the body is composed - rather than on the 75 percent that is water. I am not in a position to argue for or against this point of view. I would however like to share some of Dr. Batmanghelidj's findings and suggestions.

1.   Water regulates all of the body's functions. Every function is monitored and pegged by the flow of water. It is the primary substance and the leading agent in routine events such as brain functioning and digestion.
2.   Water distribution assures the transport of hormones, chemical messengers and nutrients to the organs.
3.   Copious amounts of water are needed for the digestion, absorption and elimination processes.
4.   When the body becomes dehydrated a water management system kicks in, a rationing and distribution system which assures that water gets to the vital organs first (brain tissues are 75+ percent water). Rationing though means that other parts of the body such as joints, do not receive the water they need for lubrication.
5.   Chronic dehydration, a persistent shortage of water established over time, leads to a deficiency disorder which causes pain and eventually leads to disease. Deficiency disorders are treated by supplementation of the missing ingredient. So that is why the treatment is to drink water.

There are no substitutes for water – not tea, not coffee, not beer or alcohol, not juice, not soup, not sodas. Herbal teas are okay, but pure water is best. You need 6-8 glasses of water a day, every day – unless you have kidney trouble or a renal disorder in which case you must consult your physician regarding water consumption.

Drink one or two glasses first thing in the morning, a half hour before you eat, and the remaining glasses throughout your day. If your urine is dark in colour it is a sign of dehydration. Joint pain is a sign of dehydration. Dyspeptic (digestive) pain is a sign of dehydration. Headaches are a sign of dehydration. Asthma and allergies are signs of dehydration. Constipation is a sign of dehydration. We are not sick says Dr. Batmanghelidj. **We are thirsty.** I think I'll go drink a glass of water.

WEEK 4
WARNING TO MEN

Okay, I may be going out on a limb here, but … I've decided to get out my silk, duvet-filled, lavender smelling boxing gloves.

No one can deny the dedication and commitment our beloved men have when it comes to taking care of their cars. Men understand about the importance of keeping their vehicles properly maintained in order to achieve maximum performance and to avoid having problems. They also know that neglecting problems can cause further damage and even result in costly repairs. Every man knows that you have to change the oil, put in new filters and top off the different fluids … in the appropriate holes. He will make an appointment for the necessary seasonal adjustments and yearly tune-ups if he can't do those himself. He will probably invest in an application of protective undercoating as well as a proper cleaning and polish. He will feel good about himself for doing what has to be done … even if it costs money - a worthy investment! Maintenance is a given; you have to do it to assure the longevity of your machine.

So why, pray tell, is it so difficult for men to take care of themselves as well as they take care of their cars? Please forgive me for being so forthright but many, if not most of you, are not taking the question of your health very seriously. Why? I am giving you time to think here. Please skip the excuses. I suspect cultural conditioning - women nurture, men provide - to be the main (unconscious) culprit. The other culprit is denial.

MYTHS
- Men are invincible. Nooo! You have to eat vegetables, exercise and take care of your health too.
- Being "healthy" takes the fun out of life. Nooo! Being sick takes the fun out of life.
- It won't happen to me. It could! As we live longer, the chances for chronic disease and ill health increase due to long-term neglect, and the accumulated negative effects of poor nutrition, lack of exercise, too much stress, as well as genetic predisposition and environmental toxins.

I am sorry. This problem of having to take responsibility for your health will not go away. You must simply accept it. Your health is entirely up to you. No two ways about it. As your Coach I must remind you to choose to eat better, drink less alcohol and smoke less, exercise more, stretch more, breathe more ... be more in touch with your feelings and your vulnerability. Only by accepting your vulnerability, will you fully embrace the need to make the necessary changes and find the courage to act. Please do. And please act before it is too late. So, go for your seasonal tune-ups and yearly check-up. Give yourself the maintenance treatment; use high-grade products and services (a worthy investment) ... don't neglect those little problems which could cause damage and result in costly repairs ... please protect the longevity of that vehicle, your body, which motors you around life.

Now ... for all you men out there making the effort to exercise, improve your eating habits or quit smoking, I give you 5 gold stars!

I wrote this article in support of all the women who have over the last 8 years, expressed their heartfelt concern about their husbands becoming ill or dying prematurely as a result of neglecting their health. This Fit Tip was originally published in February of 2008. The topic is still current. So long for now ... with love.

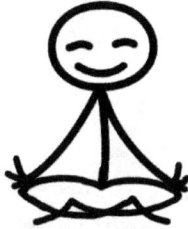

MONTH TWO
Challenge of the Month: MEDITATION

Sit quietly and in stillness for 5 – 10 minutes

What is meditation?
Meditation is a means of transforming the mind. It encourages and develops concentration, clarity, emotional positivity, and a calm seeing of the true nature of things. With regular practice you learn about the patterns and habits of your mind. You learn that you can be the master of your mind. Focused states of mind can deepen into profoundly peaceful and energized states of mind. Such experiences can have a transformative effect and can lead to a new understanding of life.
www.thebuddhistcentre.com

Here are some suggestions to help you meet the meditation challenge:
1. Try this breathing meditation: Breathe in through the nose for 3 counts, exhale through the nose for 4 counts.
Repeat 10 times.
2. Download a free Meditation app
3. Listen to Deva Premal & Miten's 21-day Mantra meditation journey which can be accessed free of charge on Spotify. www.spotify.com
4. Use prayer as a form of meditation.

WEEK 1
STILLING AND DISTILLING

This month we are going to practise integrating 5 - 10 minutes of meditation as part of our first-thing-in-the-morning (FTM) routine. We will be using this quiet moment to gently discipline and train our minds. Scientists tell us that being able to put our attention where we want, when we want, is one of the keys to optimal living and happiness. It has been my experience that this is true. Neuroscientists have discovered that when you ask the brain to meditate, it gets better not just at meditating, but at a wide range of self-control skills, including attention, focus, stress management, impulse control, and self-awareness. You can make yourself miserable or happy by the way you respond to events. Stress isn't something "out there" that needs to be controlled. Rather, it's a function of how we live, think and feel. This is what we will be tackling this month.

Please do not feel overwhelmed or threatened by this challenge. Relax with this idea. Notice if you have any resistance. If so, why? What is it? Don't give up before you start. I'm going to make it simple for you. First, commit 100 percent to doing this every day for a month. Recommit when you miss a day. Yes you can. And, you will be amazed at the brand new person you become!

Helpful tips:
1. Get comfortable - sit with dignity (in a chair is fine), tall, relaxed and with alert awareness.
2. Sit at the same time and in the same place every day to trigger a quiet mental headspace, to create a good habit.
3. Start small – 1 minute if you must, use a timer or one of the many apps available (simply google free meditation apps). Add a minute every day or so until you get to 5 minutes, etc.
4. Use anchors in your practice to keep your mind from drifting. An anchor can be anything from silently repeating a prayer or mantra, to following your breath, counting down from 10, or listening to tranquil music. Bring your attention back from thinking, back to your anchor again and again and again. Your mind will wander. That is normal. Bringing it back is how you train the mind to focus, concentrate and let go.

Over time, with consistent practice you will become more skillful. Be aware of the sensations, thoughts and emotions that arise. They are about you. Return to your breath to anchor your mind in the present moment, where what you are doing is being silent and still.

5. Don't judge your meditation. Don't get impatient with yourself. Just show up day in and day out. Meditation is a relationship with yourself, a stilling and distilling of the mind, an opportunity to make friends with yourself, to accept yourself and the way things are.

Let's do it together. After you drink your cup of warm lemon water and before you turn on any devices (iPhone, iPad, computer, radio, TV etc.), sit down in a quiet, comfortable place and practise being calm and peaceful. In so doing, as if by magic, you will improve the quality of your life.

WEEK 2
LOSING WEIGHT

I have decided to keep my boxing gloves on again this month and try to go some rounds with that gnarly, tenacious and annoying opponent: Weight Loss (WL). Oh, I can see the eyes rolling, hear the sighs and see the signs of defeat in slumped shoulders ... So Lisa, you say, how can I win that battle?

After reflection and much studying, I have settled on a radical (for boxing) and unpredictable strategy. Believe it or not, I have chosen to drop the fight. Yes, drop the fight and make friends with my opponent WL. I suggest that you do too. Struggle, stress, guilt, and low self-esteem are very detrimental to your well-being. They will adversely affect your metabolism (digestion, absorption and elimination) which is crucial to weight loss. Not only that, they will make you unhappy.

The good news about weight loss is that dieting is out and lifestyle change is in! Studies reveal that dieting, more often than not, leads to weight gain once the diet is over. So kick dieting out the door and embrace a lifestyle change which will allow you to eat, enjoy and be healthy. Sounds great! Sounds easy ... and it is, depending on your commitment to making the necessary changes.

I recommend that you read about nutrition to improve your knowledge and understanding of the body and to familiarize yourself with the many convincing health-related facts that will encourage and motivate you to make these changes.

Give your metabolism a helping hand:
- **Eat whole, real, unprocessed food** as close to its natural state as possible. A shift from refined carbohydrates such as bread, pasta, rice and sugar, in all its forms, to good carbs such as vegetables, beans, whole grains and fruit will not only help you to lose weight, but will also help to protect you against the diseases of aging and obesity.
- **Whole foods are rich in fibre.** Fibre is a powerful substance which helps you lose weight, lower your blood sugar and cholesterol; reduce your risk of cancer, heart disease and type 2 diabetes, as well as reduce inflammation.

- **Choose carbs that have a low glycemic load.** You will feel healthier and lose weight faster.
- **Reduce your portions.** Eat less and enjoy healthy snacks between meals. Spread your food intake and calories throughout the day. Eat breakfast and have your last meal at least 2 – 3 hours before going to sleep.
- **Eat slowly and enjoy your meal.** Taste, chew, swallow and be present while you eat. Create pleasure around mealtime.
- **Exercise regularly.** Walk more … how about after dinner? Use the stairs. Go to a ftness class or the gym, garden, bike or swim, etc.
- **Identify your frustrations.** Make a list. Address them by making decisions and finding solutions. Do the mouth mudra and lift the corners of your lips (smile).

If you follow these tips, you will feel more satisfied, less hungry and better nourished. You will lose weight and improve your metabolism. Try it … for more than one week … it's forever!
Yes you can! Bon Gusto.

WEEK 3
EMBRACING LIFESTYLE CHANGES

According to Roger Walsh, MD, PhD, professor of psychiatry and human behaviour at the University of California at Irvine, "Therapeutic lifestyle changes can be effective, inexpensive and enjoyable, with fewer side effects and complications than medications. In the 21st century, therapeutic lifestyles may need to be a central focus of mental, medical and public health." Science-backed research now proves that lifestyle choices profoundly affect health.

The first step in adopting a healthy lifestyle is to become self-aware; self-aware of what you eat, what you do, what you think. Self-awareness invites you to be in touch with your body (listen), to become informed (learn) and to take action (do). You can no longer pretend that you do not know what to do.

Aging and its effects on the body are inevitable, but how you age is not! That is a most powerful reason for adopting a healthy lifestyle and embracing the efforts necessary for making those changes. Your health is your most important asset. So what are you waiting for?

Tips for making lifestyle changes:
1. Be aware of what you eat, what you do or do not do and what you believe.
2. Make change by making healthy choices.
3. Set an attainable objective i.e. quit smoking, cut out fast food, stop complaining.
4. Make a plan, rally support i.e. join a fitness class, walk after dinner, find a fitness partner.
5. Take action on a daily basis because small efforts add up.
6. Don't give up. Every day is a chance to start again in some simple way.
7. Get a pedometer. Try to take 10,000 steps every day.
8. Volunteer. Cultivate meaning in your life.
9. Participate in group activities. Share your knowledge.
10. Breathe consciously, relax and enjoy. Every day.

At around 40, you suddenly realize that you can no longer get away with ignoring the issue of your health. You begin to feel the first symptoms of pain and dis – ease, which are the result of too much stress, too much wear and tear, and not enough balanced exercise and wholesome food. This pain and dis - ease signify that your cells are beginning to suffer from deficiencies in vitamins, minerals, phytonutrients and essential fatty acids. They are also showing the effects of an accumulation of stress hormones, toxins and fat cells. Chronic disease does not just fall out of the sky! The degeneration of your different body parts (joints, bones, organs, heart and blood vessels, muscles, skin, eyes, etc.) is caused by the accumulation of these deficiencies and the resulting system imbalances.

The good news? The body is designed to heal itself. Without the building blocks of good nutrition, adequate exercise and a constructive mental outlook though, the body's ability to do so is impaired. Lifestyle changes then, with regard to diet, exercise, attitude and stress management are the pillars of prevention. Don't take your health for granted! Take action now before chronic disease sets in. Take action now and manage whatever symptoms you may have. Take action now and cultivate vibrant good health to support you through the different phases of the aging process. It is never too late to start! Many of my clients have remarked that they feel better now at 60 (since they started exercising on a regular basis) than they did at 45! And that is the truth. Make a conscious choice for positive change. Embrace a lifestyle change.

WEEK 4
MY LAMENT

Okay here it goes, "The weather sucks this summer! It is absolutely lousy." There I said it. I don't know about you but I can feel the edge of frustration, irritation and annoyance colouring my frame of mind. I swear that each time I have gone kayaking on Monday and Wednesday nights it has been pouring rain. ENOUGH RAIN ALREADY. Please, please, please let the sun shine.

Dan says to me with great determination, "I'm going - rain or not!" Gotta love Dan. You know what I heard in my garden the other morning? The daylilies screaming "Throw us a life jacket. We're drowning."

My rational self is saying that it's a wet year ... La Nina you know ... the Great Lakes need it ...the water tables need it and it doesn't promote the growth of Blue Algae. My emotional self is crying and screaming, down on her knees, hands clasped to her breast, praying for sun. My conscious self reminds me to be in the present moment and accept the way things are. My Yoga teacher self is encouraging me to be grateful for my life and to find "the sun within" ... humph!

I have to admit that all my selves have a good point. Sigh ... such turmoil over the weather! How Canadian. Yet, it's not all in my head. Real physical factors are affecting my health and mood - and it's not called menopause! It's simply the lack of sunshine and "fun in the sun". Sunlight produces such deep relaxation and soothes the soul. I am yearning for sunlight, blue sky and a real summer.

Ahh, the pursuit of balance and personal happiness. If it's not one thing, it's another. We are continually working on balance: balancing our emotions, our minds and our bodies in the context of work, family, time, ambition, environmental issues, political issues, financial and economic issues, health issues. It's remarkable that we manage at all!

My Yoga teacher self invites me to calm down, to breathe, to do the mouth mudra (smile) and to be happy ... to remember how much fun I had anyway kayaking in the rain or walking with my friends in the warm cloudy, grey. And hey, what about that midnight sauna adventure - to be warm enough to go swimming in the lake - on the full moon in July? lol

Yes, I have had beautiful summer days. And yes, I have had to make a bigger effort than other summers. I am determined though, even when I get totally fed up with the weather (especially if it ruins my big party), to adjust my attitude, get out, be active and enjoy my summer – rain or shine.

To finish, thank you for your patience with my lament and for bearing witness to this stream-of-consciousness hunt for inner peace and balance. Keep up the good cheer. Namaste - the light in me honours the light in you ... and the sunlight too.

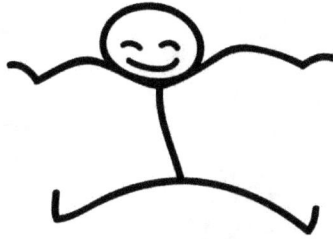

MONTH THREE
Challenge of the Month: GET MOVING

Do 15 to 20 minutes of Physical Activity

N.B. If you can't do your physical activity, first thing in the morning, do it more or less at the same time every day. The advantage of doing it first thing in the morning is that you get it done (especially if you have a busy schedule), it gets your energy moving and it makes you feel great. TRY IT.

Physical Activity suggestions:
1. Walk (the dog!)– the benefits of fresh air are immeasurable.
2. Do Qigong or Yoga.
3. Do exercises and stretching for back health.
4. Do the exercises recommended by your physiotherapist.

WEEK 1
GET MOVING

Of course, I would never ask you to do something that I do not do. As a result I now have a morning routine/ritual which I developed by gradually layering in a new healthy lifestyle habit every month, over the last three months. To be truthful, I never had a morning ritual before. I am astounded by the results! My life has changed. I am more balanced, more focused, much more productive.

Drink a cup of warm water mixed with the juice of half a lemon first thing in the morning. This hydrates and nourishes the body with essential nutrients. Next spend 5 - 10 minutes stilling your mind and body. Use music, meditation apps, prayer, whatever works for you. This is to center and ground yourself so that you can meet your day with peace and a clearer frame of mind. This month's challenge: add 20 minutes of physical activity to your morning routine.

I go for a brisk walk uphill, rain or shine, and then a swim in the lake. I feel invigorated from the walk, the fresh air and the cold water. How do I fit it in you ask? I get up half an hour earlier. I feel very satisfied with myself for having accomplished so much by 8 am. It seems to release me from the pressure of having to get things done. As a result I get a lot more done, with less effort. Every day. The cumulative effect of the three habits far outshines doing just one or two. That is my discovery.

Now if I don't start with the water I feel like something is missing, especially after a party night. The meditation, which I do for 15 minutes, seems to root me into a deeper source of energy, one not troubled by an anxious, nervous system. The walking gets my circulation going and when it is raining I rediscover the young girl in me who loved to play in the rain. Some mornings I open the door and set off at a run. These changes are organic. They are the result of augmenting my vitality, little by little. Your turn now. For those of you already doing it, 10 gold stars.

Practical tips:
- If you can't walk, for whatever reason, try to stand up every 20 minutes to counter the negative effects of sitting. If you can't stand, move your body by bending, twisting, pushing, reaching in all directions. Moving your body against gravity

procures health benefits. Accumulate your minutes gradually throughout the day.

- If you already walk, swim or bike change it up by adding a small challenge such as walking faster, including hills or varying your swim stroke. By the way if you have sore knees or hips, the water is a great place to exercise.

- If 20 minutes is too much at one time, work your way up gradually, minute by minute if necessary, or divide your time into 2 or 3 sessions. Use the walker, the cane or a walking stick if you have trouble with your balance. Get up and get going. You will be astounded at how your life changes. Don't believe me. Try it.

Two-thirds of Canadians do not meet the recommended minimum of 150 minutes a week of physical activity for health benefits. Similar stats exist for the U.S. That's twenty-five minutes a day to help prevent the onset of chronic disease, increase your vitality and improve your quality of life. Let's do this together. Establish a morning ritual and transform your life.

WEEK 2
A HEALTHY HEART

We humans have an amazing propensity for denial. Denial though can have dire consequences. Don't stick your head in the sand! Take heart in your heart health. Your loved ones will be grateful.

In Canada 90 percent of heart attacks result from coronary disease, and in the U.S. coronary artery disease is the most common type of heart disease. Coronary heart disease is a leading cause of death in North America and causes atherosclerosis, which is a narrowing of the coronary arteries due to fatty deposits called plaque. This narrowing blocks the flow of blood, nutrients and oxygen to the heart. This blockage can lead to angina (chest pain) and heart attacks. Blood clots can more easily get caught in the arteries and thus further reduce the flow of blood to the heart, and even cause death.

The good news is that coronary heart disease (CHD) is the most preventable type. A major study by the Canadian Institute of Health Research found that integrated lifestyle changes can reduce the risk by 80 percent. WOW! Both genders are equally at risk. For women the chances increase four times after menopause. So, outsmart yourself and take preventive action now!

- **Quit smoking** – This is the single most effective thing you can do for your heart. Smoking robs the heart of oxygen by accelerating the deposit of plaque in the arteries. Narrower, less elastic arteries make the heart work harder. Many people have managed to quit. So can you!

- **Exercise** – Being inactive is high on the list of major contributors to heart disease. Physically active people have half the risk of coronary heart disease than sedentary people and are 35 percent - 50 percent less likely to develop hypertension. Exercise reduces LDL cholesterol (the bad kind of fatty deposits whose accumulation causes a narrowing of the arteries) and raises HDL cholesterol (the heart-healthy type that sweeps LDL away.) Exercise strengthens the heart and helps you to maintain a healthier weight and blood pressure. The Heart and Stroke Foundation recommends 30 – 45 minutes of exercice a day. Don't despair! Accumulate: 10 minutes here, 15 minutes there ...

- **Banish belly fat** – Fat stored around the belly increases the risk of heart disease. Visceral fat lies deep within the body and releases harmful chemicals into the blood. A 15 percent decrease in total weight cuts visceral fat by as much as 41 percent. (Get to it!) Your waist-to-hip ratio (WHR) will help determine if you are carrying too much dangerous belly fat. Measure your waist at its smallest point, in inches, and then measure your hips at their widest point. Divide your waist measurement by your hip measurement. A WHR of .85 and over in women and more than .9 in men is strongly linked to an increased risk heart disease. Go on, get out the measuring tape and look the truth in the eye. Take action if necessary.

- **Keep tabs on your blood pressure** – High blood pressure forces your heart to work even harder and may cause it to become thick and stiff. Lowering blood pressure to acceptable levels can reduce heart attacks by an average of 20 percent to 50 percent. Exercise helps to lower blood pressure; medication controls it. Don't fool around with blood pressure. Consult your doctor. Get tested. Uncontrolled high blood pressure is known as the silent killer.

- **Eat heart smart** – Eat high-fibre, cholesterol-lowering foods such as whole grains, legumes, nuts and seeds, deep coloured fish containing heart-protective marine Omega-3 fatty acids. Limit refined, processed foods. Eat plenty of raw fresh fruit and vegetables for their vitamins, minerals and antioxidants. Limit salt and booze. Oh well, you gotta do what you gotta do … and I know you can. (You will feel so much better.)

- **Deal with diabetes** - Up to 80 percent of people with diabetes die as a result of a heart attack or stroke, and diabetic women face a threefold risk of a heart attack. The persistent high blood sugar levels of diabetes damage arteries and small blood vessels and accelerate artery-plugging atherosclerosis. If you have diabetes, modify your other cardiac risk factors: smoking, lack of exercise, high blood pressure, excess weight and high cholesterol. Have a diabetes check-up every three months and a full evaluation once a year. If you don't have diabetes but are 40 or older, get your blood sugar levels checked soon and, thereafter, every three years—especially if you have a high body mass index, high blood pressure, elevated cholesterol or a family history of diabetes.

- **Brush up on oral hygiene** - Two of the cheapest defensive weapons are your toothbrush and dental floss. One study of Canadians (aged 36 to 69) found that those with severe gum disease (known also as periodontal disease) were three to seven times more at risk for fatal heart disease. Bacteria entering the bloodstream from the mouth can invade the heart. These microbes may promote artery-damaging inflammation as well as contribute to clot formation by binding to the fatty deposits in arteries.

My healthy heart tip to you is: open your heart to laughter, to life and to loving. Boom, boom.

These tips are from the article Have a Heart by Michele Sponagle, Canadian Health and lifestyle magazine, Fall, 2006.

WEEK 3
THE PHYSIOLOGY OF AGING

Brace yourself. Today, I am going to share with you some facts about aging. They say ignorance is bliss, but I beg to differ. Too many of you are still going about complaining over this ache and that pain, swallowing this pill and conveniently chalking it up to "aging". Well, yes, and no! YES, because aging is in part responsible for the trouble. And, NO, because there are many concrete actions we can take to slow down the process of aging and to keep us feeling "young".

So here it goes:

1. At around 35 years of age we begin to lose 1 percent of our bone mass per year. Osteoporosis is a disease related to loss of bone mass.

2. Loss of flexibility starts at around 35 years of age as well and leads to decreased range of motion, pain and rigidity which eventually affect mobility. The body must move in order to remain healthy.

3. At 45 to 50 years of age muscle mass begins to decline by 3 kg per decade. This decline is due to a decrease in growth hormone production and a lack of physical activity.

4. Body fat increases in relation to muscle loss because muscle burns more calories at rest than fat does. This fact alone leads to weight gain and increases the challenge of maintaining a healthy weight. Accumulated fat is deposited around the vital organs, which increases the risk for heart disease. Fat is a storage house for the harmful toxins the body cannot eliminate. The more toxins you have stored in your body the more at risk you are for disease, and the harder it is to lose weight. Are you getting depressed yet?

5. The structure of the blood vessels of the heart changes due to the increased rigidity of the vessel walls and accumulated LDLs (bad cholesterol). These changes cause both blood pressure and blockage problems which increase the chances of heart disease.

6. With aging the cardiovascular system becomes less sensitive to neurological stimulation. This causes a decrease in heart rate, blood pressure reflex time as well as blood flow to the

muscles. This slows both the output capacity and recovery time. Stop Lisa. Enough!

7. No, there is more. How about posture, lung health, balance, memory, eyes, ears and skin! Need I go into more detail? Are you ready to give up, roll over and die right now? No wait! I have solutions.

Here are Health Canada's physical activity recommendations to help reduce the risk of chronic disease, increase autonomy and improve quality of life:

1. **Endurance exercise:** 4 to 7 times a week for cardiovascular health.
2. **Strength and balance training:** 2 to 3 times a week for weight maintenance, better posture, prevention of osteoporosis and maintaining autonomy.
3. **Stretching:** daily for pain relief and maintaining suppleness.

Many of you already do some form of physical activity every week. But is your routine balanced? Here are some suggestions.

Walkers and bike riders: whole body stretching (neck, shoulders, back and legs – warm up before and stretch after), interval training (alternate between intensity and rest), upper body and core strengthening, attention to posture (bad posture creates an imbalance in muscle tone which in turn causes wear and tear on the joints).

Gardeners and yard workers: whole body stretching (twists, swings, forward and side bends, neck, shoulder and wrist rotations plus squats – stretch before, during and after), attention to posture and proper lifting techniques as well as endurance exercises (walking, biking, swimming) for your cardio-vascular health.

Construction workers: whole body stretching (twists, swings, forward and side bends, neck and shoulder rotations – before and after), attention to posture and proper lifting techniques, relaxation (massage and sauna) and Yoga to release accumulated muscle tension.

Kayaking and canoeing: whole body stretching (shoulder, neck, back and leg stretching – before and after), lower body and core strengthening, attention to posture.

Shoulder issues, tendonitis, bursitis: avoid weight bearing and painful range of motion on the injured side. Do the physical therapy exercises prescribed to you. Do endurance and balance training, strengthen the legs and the core as well as gentle stretching of the upper body, back and legs.

Hip, knee and feet issues: do the physical therapy exercises prescribed; exercise free of pain in the pool, on a recumbent bicycle or on a mat (reduce range of motion and weight bearing); do gentle stretching and wear good shoes.

Back pain, Arthritis and Fibromyalgia: gentle "lubricating" range of motion movements and strengthening (Lisa's Chair Program DVD and Back Pain DVD, Swimming, Qigong); reduce range of motion and take time for relaxation. www.agesmartfitness.com/store/

Overweightness: strength training, daily endurance training such as walking and swimming with an interval approach (alternating between effort and rest); work with a partner.

There are three dimensions to human frailty – time, disease and disuse. You can't do much about time, disease is very challenging but, with regard to disuse, you have the power to make positive change. The ball is in your court. Are you game? Just do it.

WEEK 4
THE GIFT OF LOVING KINDNESS

Imagine if you had the power to set everything right! And if you did, what would that be? Save the planet, reverse global warming, clean the water and the air? Eradicate poverty? Provide education and food for everyone! Put an end to terrorism, religious fanaticism and WAR! Abolish corruption and greed. Find a cure for AIDS. That would be a good start. Find peaceful solutions for the problems of racism, intolerance and bigotry. Dignity for all human beings! Free Tibet and all other countries and people under siege! **Imagine** how incredible that would be. Equality for the sexes! Safe harbours for all children. An end to slave labour, forced prostitution, sexual aberrations, drug addiction, alcoholism and violent crimes. Just thinking about it makes me feel giddy. The overwhelming nature of the task also makes me feel sad, angry, doubtful, numb ... yet determined to act no matter how small my contribution may be.

One of the challenging ideas that I have come across in my quest for spiritual growth is this: if you want others to change, you must first change yourself. I love this challenge because it motivates me to self-responsibility and conscious action. If I want change I have to get involved. I have to commit to making a personal moral effort, to having a correct attitude of mind and to making progress in what is right. This challenge calls forward the best in human nature, and by doing so, sets up the conditions for positive influence to emanate from good example. The logic behind this idea becomes very compelling when you grasp the cumulative effect that self-responsibility, conscious action and positive influence can have on your personal life, your community and your world. **Imagine** one by one by one setting in motion a wave of compassion ... a gentle, adapting and penetrating swell of loving kindness and positive action growing ever bigger.

I first came across the concept of Maitri or "loving kindness" (the translation of the Sanskrit word Maitri) in 1985 when I was doing my Masters degree in Dance Therapy at Naropa Institute in Boulder, Colorado. This ancient Tibetan concept (to summarize in an overly simplistic fashion) reminds us that we need to act with "loving kindness" toward ourselves in order to manage the problems and neuroses created by the basic human drives of passion, ignorance and aggression.

Experiencing loving kindness towards yourself opens the door to acceptance and forgiveness, to overcoming shame and guilt, to releasing pain and fear; to freeing yourself of suffering so that you can act with loving kindness towards others. Maitri changed my life and gradually set me free to have the courage to love, to be kind and to care. **Imagine.**

My wish for all of us is that we can bathe in the warm waters of loving kindness and that the healing balm of loving kindness will embrace and envelope our deep selves, our families, our neighbours, our communities and our troubled, off-kiltered world. I wish for us to cultivate gratitude and temperance, to grow in our understanding that through the small gesture of making positive change in ourselves, we are contributing to positive global change for our children's children and their children.

In the words of John Lennon *"Imagine all the people, living life in peace. You may say that I'm a dreamer, but I am not the only one. I hope someday you'll join us and the world will live as one."* I'm in. How about you?

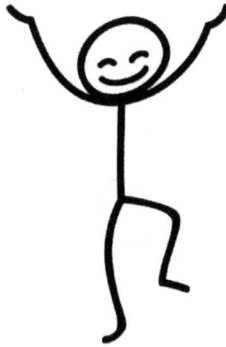

MONTH FOUR
Challenge of the Month: DISCIPLINE

Practice being disciplined. Continue your FTM
(First-Thing-in-the-Morning) routine

Suggestions:
Choose one thing to be disciplined about every week in the area of
either diet, mental attitude or physical activity. And do it.

Examples:
- reduce your portions
- do not buy any chips or soda this week
- have dessert only on the weekend
- do not eat any wheat this week
- use the stairs
- go for a walk after dinner
- focus on things which make you happy

WEEK 1
THE D WORD!

The D word. Can you guess what it is? DISCIPLINE. Right! I can hear the silent groans, see the guilty looks. We have been working on integrating a different healthy habit per month, for the last three months. Step 1: Drink a cup of warm water mixed with the juice of half a lemon, first thing in the morning. Step 2: Be still and quiet (meditation) for 5 to 10 minutes. Step 3: Do 20 minutes of physical activity - your choice. Practising discipline is this month's challenge.

Why is it that so many of us find being disciplined difficult? Willpower in itself is a very limited resource. When you rely on willpower alone it tends to reinforce defeat rather than success. The problem is not in the intention or desire for change, but in the set-up. Discipline requires strategy to achieve success. You have to choose it. Plan for it. Do it, no matter what. Some mornings I don't feel like doing my FTM (first-thing-in-the-morning) routine. From experience though I know that as soon as I am out the door I will be enjoying myself and feeling fantastic. So, the discipline is not about doing my routine - big effort in my mind but rather about getting out the door – little manageable effort.

Here are a few practical tips to help you set up for being disciplined:
1. Commit 100 percent to the habit for at least 4 weeks. Then recommit. This is the key to your success.
2. Be realistic. Write it down. Start with things you like and are easy for you.
3. Break your challenge down into steps. Go one step at a time. Let the routine carry you forward.
4. Practise at the same time, in the same place and in a similar way every day to help set up your routine and "wire in" your new lifestyle habit(s).
5. Get out the door! Don't make a mountain out of a molehill.
6. You don't have to be great at it every day, but do it every day.

Here are a few signs that your efforts are paying off:
• You have more energy.
• You feel healthier, calmer, more focused.

- What was difficult is becoming easier.
- You notice changes in your body, your mind and in your overall state of balance.
- You feel satisfaction and pride in yourself.
- You are more productive, can handle stress better.
- You feel stronger, you naturally want to do more, add variety and challenge.
- You sleep more peacefully.

Discipline is the practice of bringing repeated attention to your intention. When you repeat an action it creates neural pathways which support your thought or behaviour patterns until they become integrated as new habits. These habits become automatic because they are wired into your brain. Discipline creates good habits which, when practised consistently, become a healthy way of life, effortlessly. Mindfully deciding what to pick as habits can change your life. Go ahead, practise being disciplined by making smart and steady choices. Change your life for the better. You can do it.

WEEK 2
CLEAN FROM THE INSIDE OUT

Clean the body from the inside out? Detoxifying and cleansing are a normal part of your body processes. The three main organs that detoxify the body are the liver, the colon and the kidneys. The liver acts as a filter preventing toxins and bacteria from passing into the bloodstream. The colon's main role is to flush out toxic chemicals before they can do you any harm. That is why we want to keep our colon flowing regularly, so the toxins don't get stuck there! The kidneys constantly filter your blood and get rid of toxins in the form of urine. Drinking water is an important support for the function of the kidneys.

Detoxification is what your body naturally does to neutralize, transform or get rid of unwanted materials or toxins. It is a primary function of the body to keep us alive and healthy. To experience vibrant health, you need to maintain these three key organs by nourishing your body with the right nutrients. A great way to support your natural detoxification system is to feed it alkalinizing and cleansing foods. Here is a list of nine such foods which you can integrate into your diet on a regular basis to give your body the tools it needs to slowly cleanse, rebuild and thrive.

Avocados: are a good source of healthy fats which help speed up the metabolism and help in weightloss. They promote healthy skin and stimulate the cleansing actions of the digestive system.

- *Cleanse Nutrients:* glutathione, fibre, antioxidants, good fats, potassium.
- *Cleanse Target:* gall bladder, digestive system

Cabbage: contains fibre, antioxidants, alkaline minerals and more good fats. It's a great all-round cleanser, powerful gastrointestinal tract cleanser and an anti-inflammatory

- *Cleanse Nutrients:* fibre, antioxidants, good fats, manganese, folate, B6 and potassium.
- *Cleanse Target:* gastrointestinal tract and digestive system

Kale: is a green leafy vegetable, a natural antioxidant and anti-inflammatory. Kale gives a big boost of chlorophyll (green) to help cleanse the blood

- *Cleanse Nutrients:* chlorophyll, antioxidants, good fats, anti-inflammatory

- *Cleanse Target:* blood, digestive system

Cucumber: is hydrating - eat it often!
- *Cleanse Nutrients:* high-alkaline water content, antioxidant, Vitamin C, B, K, manganese, copper and potassium, fibre
- *Cleanse Target:* liver.

Spinach: is one of the most nutritious and alkaline vegetables you can eat.
- *Cleanse Nutrients:* fibre, chlorophyll, antioxidants, anti-inflammatory, anti-carcinogenic.
- *Cleanse Target:* blood and colon.

Broccoli: part of the cruciferous family and renowned for its cancer-fighting properties. Supports the digestive and cardiovascular systems.
- *Cleanse Nutrients:* critical detoxifying phytonutrients, fibre, antioxidants, anti-inflammatory, anti-carcinogenic.
- *Cleanse Target:* digestive system.

Celery: easy to use in juices, soups, salads, snacks. Kids love it.
- *Cleanse Nutrients:* fibre, antioxidants anti-inflammatory, good fats, manganese, folate, B6 and potassium.
- *Cleanse Target:* GI tract and digestive system.

Ginger: is an anti-oxidant that helps to increase the movement of food through the intestines, boosts the immune system and calms the stomach. It is great in juices and smoothies, to spice up stir fries or to drink as a tea
- *Cleanse Nutrients:* anti-inflammatory, anti-septic, anti-carcinogenic.
- *Cleanse Target:* intestines and digestive tract.

Garlic: is an anti-inflammatory - eat it every day!
- *Cleanse Nutrients:* manganese, sulphur compounds, anti-inflammatory.
- *Cleanse Target:* liver, immune system.

To improve your results, buy organic and eat foods raw or lightly steamed. Drink plenty (8 glasses a day) of fresh water. Sweating is another way the body eliminates toxins. A little knowledge can go a long way when it is supported by action on a daily basis. Enjoy these delicious and healthy foods as you become more vibrant, energized and slim! Attain health through food not pills!

WEEK 3
RESILIENCE

It's amazing the resilience of the human spirit isn't it? Think back on your own life, on the challenges you or others you know, have had to face. Challenges come in varying degrees of difficulty and intensity. Resilience is the ability to become strong, healthy, or successful again after something bad happens. How resilient are you? New scientific research shows that there are four types of resilience we can work on and develop our strengths in. They are Physical, Mental, Emotional and Social Resilience. We can actually build our resilience by doing some very simple things. Would you like to know what they are? Let me tell you.

1. **Physical Resilience:** *Never sit still for more than one hour at a time.* You don't have to be a super star athlete. Just get up and move around. It creates momentum. Once you get your energy moving, it keeps you moving.

2. **Mental Resilience:** *Tackle tiny goals regularly to boost your willpower.* Why tiny, because you know you can be successful. Puzzles, games, new hobbies. Read books, travel. Keep your mind stimulated.

3. **Emotional Resilience:** *3:1 positive emotion ratio.* Experiencing three positive emotions for every negative emotion will dramatically improve your health and your ability to successfully undertake any problem you are facing.

4. **Social Resilience:** *Reach out to one person you care for every day.* This is the way we get strength from our family, our neighbours, our friends and our community. Another great way is through gratitude and touch.

Science shows that people who regularly boost their Physical, Mental, Emotional and Social resilience live 10 years longer than everyone else! It is remarkable how little feats, simple, easy, little feats can have such a profound impact on what you feel and how you live. I guess the key in all of this life is to understand that the power lies within you. The power is in your hands to create the life that you want to live, merely by doing simple little things on a regular basis. It has been proven to add years to your life.

So what's it going to take to make the difference in your own life? What's it going to take for you to accept to be the master of your life? I guess, really, the first place to start is to make a commitment to yourself. You can do it. You can give that love to yourself. You can be courageous. You can do the simple little things like reach out to one person every day that you care about, to share a kind word or give a hug - 6 seconds is all it takes to raise your level of Oxytocin, the trust and social bonding hormone. There is no room for judgement here. There is only room for encouragement; to encourage you to use the tools, as many of them as possible, to change your life for the better. I believe in you. Yes I do!

WEEK 4
AWAKE TO LIFE

I don't know about you but I am "jonesin'" for some green! Green, green, green … green grass, tender spring-green leaves, green plants with yellow, pink, red, orange, purple, blue and white flowers. Vibrant life-force green. Heart Chakra green. Green for the environment.

It's coming. The smell of spring has begun to titillate my nose. My ears rejoice to hear song birds sing. My eyes delight in the lengthening of the day and my body/mind is uplifted by it. I feel a surge of energy flowing through me like the sap flowing in the Maple trees. Can you feel it too... this passionate awakening of life? Close your eyes. Still your mind. Connect. Spring is in the air. It's time for renewal.

Breathe in deeply. Breathe out. Take note of your surroundings. Appreciate the beauty that is before your eyes. Be grateful for your life. Count your blessings. Choose life. New beginnings are at hand. Nature is preparing to burst into life as it plays out its age-old role in the Cycle of Life.

Sun. Wind. Rain. Run-off and mud. Yes, the melt may be troublesome, very troublesome. Some years are like that - difficult. It is part of the human journey and it is common to us all. Unbidden, life bestows on each and every one of us challenges which test our strength, our resilience and our power to heal. This has recently occurred in our community*. Here too new beginnings are at hand.

Although we have been shaken and brusquely reminded of our fragility, we have also been awakened to life. How easily we get caught up and take for granted this precious gift! Undeniably, life's journey is so very hard sometimes. And yet the journey is filled with so much beauty, so many pleasures of all kinds, of all flavours, of magnificent sights to behold, discoveries to be made and a myriad of sensations to experience and enjoy.

There are times when we must allow ourselves to be softened, to be opened, even to be broken apart in order to blossom back into life like a beautiful spring flower. I extend my deepest condolences to all concerned and invite everyone to honour the departed by celebrating life on a daily basis.

* 2009 *The roof of the Gourmet Du Village warehouse collapsed in killing 3 women.*

REFLECTION
DON'T GIVE UP!

Don't feel bad. No one has 100 percent success everyday when they attempt to make changes. We all lapse back into our old ways at some point or another because these old ways are connected to our emotions, to our beliefs, to our level of stress and to our unconscious patterns. If any of these aspects get out of balance they immediately trigger our weaknesses and bad habits.

So, and this is critical, don't give up just because you have had a relapse for a few days, or because you feel bad. Don't use that as an excuse to give up. Just start again and continue the best that you can day in, day out. Perseverance will become your new benchmark for success; did I take action today? The more conscious and proactive you are in this process, the better will be your progress and success. Each little step adds up and in no time you will have advanced in leaps and bounds. Remember every time you accomplish your goals you empower yourself and, in so doing, become a creative force in your own life. Now that's exciting.

The recipe is simple: a little exercise, good nutritious food and a time for stillness every day. Roll up your sleeves; make judicious choices and go for it! 10 Gold Stars for making it to here!

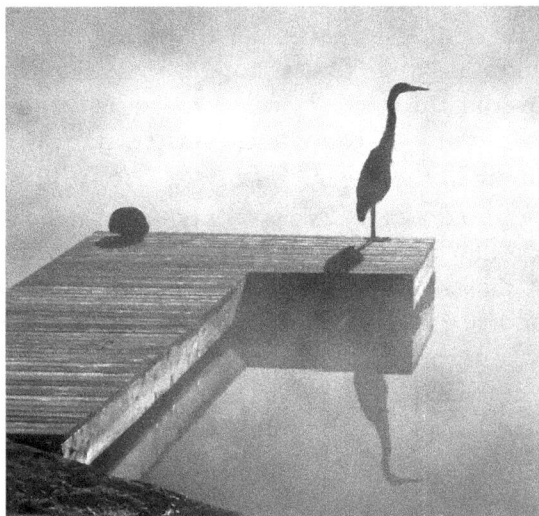

PART TWO
THE INWARD JOURNEY

"You gain strength, courage and confidence by every experience in which you really stop to look fear in the face.
Do the thing you think you cannot do".

Eleanor Roosevelt

INVITATION
LIFE'S A TRIP

My Mom has said that as she gets older the years seem to go by faster and faster. Could it be true? I guess some years you're happy that the year is finally over because, let's face it, some years are just plain awful. Hardship, illness, injury, unhappiness, disaster, tragedy, oh cruel life. As they used to say in the late 60s, *"Life's a Trip."* Oh yeah and there was also *"Keep on Truckin'!"* Now we say, *"Life is a Journey."* And so it is, so it is. All in all I have had both. Bad years in which I learned so much about myself, about life, about choices and action, or non-action. And good years, where the sun shone gloriously in my life and illuminated my way to a joyful heart. In retrospect I fully appreciate my fifty-five years of experience – the good and the bad. I suppose it is the maturity I have acquired, the ability to better handle my emotions as well as my improved perspective on life, my better understanding of humans (now that takes time). Also, all the practical, down-to-earth experience of living with its myriad of responsibilities, challenges and state of affairs to manage: kids, house, car, work, money, relationships, family, hobbies, along with social, economic and political realities. And we have the great good fortune of living in a safe democracy which, no matter how flawed, provides a better quality of life than most places on earth.

This year we are fortunate; no stock market crash (although the economic portrait is still shaky), no life-threatening virus (funny how we no longer hear anything about our friend H1N1- disappeared right off the face of the earth!). Still, the planet is deeply troubled, off kilter. I don't know about you but I just can't buy into this whole commercial thing. The stress, the expense, the illusions, the waste. No. I prefer real things like love and sharing peace and joy. I am a sucker for that warm, fuzzy feeling. I like presents too. Homemade presents. Presents from the heart. Gifts of kindness. The most important presents (presence) are forgiveness and acceptance. By letting go of hurt and anger we open the way to love which is the greatest gift of all. I know. I sound corny. But I am sure many of you out there catch my drift (isn't that from the 60s too?) Love thyself, love thy neighbour, love thy planet. Here we go, the inward journey.

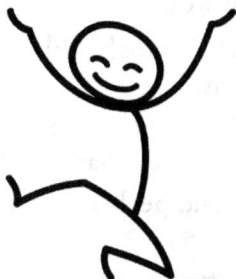

MONTH FIVE
Challenge of the Month: EAT YOUR GREENS

Make a green juice or smoothie. If you can't juice then make
sure you eat your greens either raw or lightly steamed
for lunch and dinner every day

Suggestions:
1. Use a blender if you don't have a juicer or magic bullet. My
   preferred time for my green juice or smoothie is around 11am.
   Find the time that is best for you. Drink it on an empty stomach.
2. Try the green juice recepies at:
   www.mindbodygreen.com/0-8155/3-yummy-green-juice-
   recipes-to-convert-skeptics.html
3. Eat dark green vegetables – kale, spinach, parsley, cucumbers,
   broccoli, rapini.
4. Eat salads made with romaine lettuce or mesclun and add a
   variety of green, red, yellow, orange and purple vegetables
5. Use organic produce as often as you can.

N.B. Raw vegetables can be difficult to digest for some. Steam them
lightly to facilitate digestion. Gradually increase the amount of vegetables to prevent digestive troubles, constipation and gas from the
sudden increase in fibre.

For those of you with digestive issues, including irritable bowel syndrome, constipation, diarrhea and acid reflux: eat fewer vegetables. Vegetables (as well as some fruits) are often high in insoluble fibre. While soluble fibre can be soothing for the gut, consuming large amounts of insoluble fibre when your gut is inflamed is a little bit like rubbing a wire brush against an open wound.

There are steps you can take to make these foods more digestible and less likely to cause problems.

1. Never eat insoluble fibre foods on an empty stomach. Always eat them with other foods that contain soluble fibre.

2. Remove the stems and peels from vegetables and fruits high in insoluble fibre.

3. Dice, mash, chop, grate or blend foods high in insoluble fibre to make them easier to break down during digestion.

4. Insoluble fibre foods are best eaten well-cooked: steamed thoroughly, boiled in soup, braised, etc. Avoid consuming them in stir-fries and if you do eat them raw, prepare them as described in #3 above.

The Dirty Dozen (full of pesticides)
Celery, Peaches, Strawberries, Apples, Domestic Blueberries, Nectarines, Sweet Bell Peppers, Spinach, Kale, Collard Greens, Cherries, Potatoes, Imported Grapes and Lettuce.

The Clean Fifteen (organic or not)
Onions, Avocados, Sweet Corn, Pineapples, Mango, Sweet Peas, Asparagus, Kiwi Fruit, Cabbage, Eggplant, Cantaloupe, Watermelon, Grapefruit, Sweet Potatoes, and Sweet Onions.

WEEK 1
THE POWER OF GREEN

Eat Your Greens. Oh no Lisa, not that! Yes my friends. Challenge of the Month no.5: **Eat Your Greens** Why? CHLOROPHYLL. Chlorophyll is the important green compound that acts as your internal healer, cleanser, antiseptic, cell stimulator, rejuvenator and red blood cell builder. The greener the leaves, the more concentrated the amount of chlorophyll. Taken consistently in sufficient amounts, chlorophyll has these powerful remedial effects:

1. Increases red blood cell counts
2. Alleviates blood sugar problems
3. Improves bowel functions
4. Reduces or eliminates body odours
5. Relieves gastric ulcers
6. Greatly relieves respiratory troubles like asthma and sinusitis
7. Detoxifies and cleanses
8. Reduces inflammation pain
9. Melts away toxic fats
10. Kills bacteria in wounds, speeds up healing
11. Soothes painful hemorrhoids
12. Improves milk production in lactating mothers

Are you surprised by all that plant greens can do for your health? It is real medicine. The single, biggest game-changer in improving my diet and gaining optimal health was to add a green juice into my daily routine. No doubt about it. My level of energy increased, my skin became more radiant, my moods more balanced. I became more resistant to illness and was better able to maintain my weight - even going through the challenges of menopause! Juicing allows us to eat a bigger variety of vegetables in bigger quantities, which in turn leaves us better hydrated, better nourished and feeling on top of the world. Green vegetable juices could be life changers for you too!

I juice with my blender rather than a juicer. I don't get as nutrient-dense a drink, but in my case my body loves the fibre. The extra fibre really makes me feel better. Dietary fibre aids in digestion, helps regulate blood sugar levels and keeps you feeling full-longer. It plays a vital role in eliminating toxins as a result of regular bowel movements.

When the blood sugar is successfully controlled and regulated, you will lose excess weight and more easily maintain a healthy body.

Getting started: I have been making this juice 5 mornings a week for 3 years now. It works for me.

Recipe:
1. Blend together 1/2 a peeled lemon, a chunk of peeled ginger, 1 stalk celery, 1/2 cucumber partially peeled (unpeeled if organic), 1/2 cup organic apple, mango or pear juice. Blend.
2. Add big handful of spinach, a handful of kale and a small handful of parsley finely chopped (easier on my old blender). Add water. Blend.
3. Dilute with more water if the juice is too thick, pour it into a mason jar (or two), and drink gradually.

This may be too radical for most of you, so here is a website for some simpler green juice ideas for beginners: www.mindbodygreen. com/0-8155/3-yummy-green-juice-recipes-to-convert-skeptics.html.

Use organic products for your juices as often as possible. I also love to make salads that are much more than lettuce leaves. I add a variety of finaly chopped raw vegetables, as well as some nuts and nutritional yeast. I then toss it with a simple vinaigrette: olive oil, organic apple cider vinegar, Bragg and finely chopped garlic. Mmmm delicious.

I hope you will join me in this Healthy Lifestyle Habits challenge and change your life for the better one little step at a time. *"Bon appétit"* as Julie Child would say.

WEEK 2
WHY FRUIT AND VEGGIES ARE SO IMPORTANT

The human body is a complex system that needs energy to carry out its metabolic processes. To maintain its functions, the body needs a constant supply of nutrients. These nutrients are **enzymes, vitamins, minerals, phytonutrients, proteins, essential fats and fibre.** They are responsible for the growth, repair and maintenance of the body. Many of these nutrients come from fresh, raw or lightly steamed fruit and vegetables.

Enzymes

We need enzymes to digest food. Enzymes convert the food we eat into a form which is easily absorbed by the blood-stream. A unique property of enzymes is that they carry the life force within them. They are living proteins that help transform and store energy. Enzymes help balance and restore the immune system and heal many diseases. Enzymes even help repair our DNA and our RNA. Enzymes are combinations of proteins, vitamins, and minerals in an active molecular form. They dissolve fibre and are anti-inflammatory.

When we cook our fruit and vegetables we destroy many of the enzymes that help us digest it. The body is then forced to use its own digestive enzymes which, over time, depletes our store of this very important nutrient that keeps us alive and healthy. Chemists are able to synthesize some of these nutrients, but they have not been able to "breathe life" into them. The "life-force factor" has never been recreated. That is why it is so important to consume raw fruit, vegetables, sprouts and nuts. Some people have trouble digesting raw vegetables. Digestive distress like gas, bloating and abdominal pain are common reactions associated with eating raw vegetables. Until your inner eco-system is healthy, you may have trouble digesting raw vegetables. To help with this problem cook your vegetables by baking, simmering, sautéing or lightly steaming them to make them more digestible.

Vitamins

Without vitamins our cells would not function properly, our organs would suffer and eventually we would no longer be able to survive. Vitamins help regulate our metabolism, help convert fat and carbohydrates into energy and assist in forming bone and tissue. Guess what happens to the vitamin content when you cook your food? A large percentage of the vitamins are destroyed. By lightly steaming your vegetables you will lose less vitamins. This will help your system adapt to digesting the cellulose fibre of raw vegetables.

Minerals

Mineral deficiencies are important factors in the cause of disease. Minerals have a synergistic relationship with vitamins. They help each other help us. Minerals are not sensitive to heat but will leach out if cooked in boiling water. Lightly steaming is the best cooking method for retaining the mineral content of fruit and vegetables.

Phytonutrients

Phytonutrients are what give fruits and vegetables their colour. Phytonutrients protect the body and fight disease. They also fight cancer and help your heart. The brighter the colour of the fruit or vegetable, the more nutrient combatants it has to prevent degenerative diseases. Phytonutrients are at the leading edge of research on nutrition. They provide medicine for cell health. Phytonutrients in freshly harvested plant foods are diminished by cooking.

"Food sustains us … Yet what we eat may affect our risk for several of the leading causes of death for Americans notably heart disease, stroke, arteriosclerosis, diabetes, some types of cancer. These disorders now account for more than two-thirds of all deaths in the United States." former Surgeon General Dr. C. Everett Koop. The numbers are similar for Canadians. As we become more mindful of what we eat, we can make choices that promote health over illness. What happens when we learn to satisfy our pleasure receptors with healthy food? Our lives improve. Eating raw or lightly steamed foods leads to improved energy, better mental focus, less aches and pains. It also helps to eliminate headaches and skin problems. I am feeding my body with what it needs to thrive, not just survive.

Remember though, raw vegetables are only a beneficial source IF you can digest them. Many people's digestive systems are simply too weak to digest the cellulose (insoluble fibre) of raw vegetables in spite of all their natural enzymes. Refer to the tips on page 52 for helpful hints.

WEEK 3
ARE YOU SITTING TOO MUCH?

Are you aware that sitting for hours on end behind a computer, in front of a TV, reading a good book or driving in traffic is really, really bad for you? Mounting research suggests that sitting, in and of itself, is a risk factor for poor health and premature death. Your body declines rapidly when sitting for long periods, even if you are very fit. Exercising as much as five times a week for a half hour to an hour each time still falls far short of optimum fitness if you sit most of the rest of the time! Who would have thought?

Dr. Joan Vernikos, former director of NASA's Life Sciences Division and author of Sitting Kills, Moving Heals, was one of the primary doctors responsible for ensuring the health of astronauts. Her research on the health ramifications of space travel proved that you get close to a 10-fold acceleration of the aging process when you live in a gravity-free environment! Chronic, uninterrupted sitting mimics a low-gravity situation; you do not exert your body against the forces of gravity. She discovered that the act of standing up is actually more effective than walking for counteracting the ill effects of sitting. The change in posture is what has the most beneficial impact on your health, not the act of standing in and of itself. The key is to repeatedly interrupt your sitting. Standing up 35 times at once will provide only a small percent of the benefit of standing up once every 20 minutes. **Get this: it is not how many hours of sitting that is bad for you, it's how often you interrupt that sitting that is GOOD for you!**

Moving against gravity stimulates our physiological functions. Lipoprotein lipase is an important enzyme that attaches to fat in your bloodstream and transports it into your muscles to be used as fuel. Lipoprotein lipase is dramatically reduced during inactivity and increases with activity. The most effective activity is to stand up from a seated position. Simply by standing up, you are actively helping your body to burn fat for fuel. Research has proven that standing up once every hour is more effective for achieving cardiovascular and metabolic changes than walking on a treadmill for 15 minutes! Go figure.

Fit Tips for countering the ill effects of prolonged sitting:
1. Stand up around 35 times over the period of a day to counteract the cardiovascular health risks associated with sitting.

2. Move (bend, reach, twist) and shift position often.

3. Program an online timer, your watch, cellphone or whatever to go off every 20 minutes. When it goes off, stand up.

4. Alternately stand up and sit down really slowly five times.

5. You can do four jump squats or four lunges to augment the exposure to gravity. Jumping up and down gets you up to six times the force of gravity.

6. If you squat and stand, you can get the maximum benefit of working against the force of gravity. By adding jumping to it (going from a squat to a jump, landing into a squat again), you end up with about 6.5 G's. Who cares what you look like at the office!

The human body is astonishing. It's never too late to reverse damage and delay aging. *So Get Up! Stand Up! Stand up for your right* ... to be healthy. You can do this. It's easy.

WEEK 4
AGING GRACEFULLY

The original title for this Tip was Old, Older, Dead. I agree, awful. Frankly I was shocked with my own mind ... and yet why was this thought welling up from my unconscious?

Of late, an 82-year-old client has been saying to me "You know Lisa, I am programmed to die." He is not being gloomy; he is just looking truth straight in the eye. Our bodies are not designed for eternal life - at least not over the course of one lifetime - and he's acutely aware of it. Aging and all the accompanying annoyances and stark realities is inevitable, as is death. Well duh Lisa, you say. But when he conveys that thought to me and also tells me about all that he used to be able to do and all that he has accomplished I almost "get it". I almost comprehend and for a brief moment, profoundly grasp how precious and magnificent my life really is.

On occasion this same client - he maintains that I am instrumental in keeping him alive - is "fighting mad" about the limitations and problems aging has "gifted" him. It might even make him swear. From Diabetes Type 2 to a quintuple heart bypass to osteoporosis, not to mention failing eyesight, poor hearing, memory loss, wrinkling, thickening of the waist and having to walk with a cane ... who can blame him? And yet to his credit he never gives up, no matter how big the hurdle, on trying to keep himself healthy. As a result he has improved his quality of life and autonomy ten fold. He achieves this by being proactive. He studies nutrition, watches his diet, takes his medications and supplements, exercises on a regular basis and keeps his mind active. He is passionate about life and living. I am the fortunate one because he imparts his wisdom and hard-earned experience to me. And I am grateful for it.

Here then are some thoughts on aging gracefully:
1. **Gratitude:** Life is good! - enjoy the moment and be thankful for beauty and all the good things in your life.
2. **Discipline:** abide in what endures such as health, family and love, and continue to lead a normal life; stay active and involved, continue to learn.
3. **Awareness:** caution and a sense of seriousness regarding your

health and aging situation will help reduce the risk of chronic disease and injury.

4. **Acceptance:** greet the changes brought on by aging with respect – no sulking; accept and honour the way things are, adapt.

5. **Appreciation:** do not take for granted your health, your youthfulness, your beauty, your abilities – relish them, you may not always be able to.

6. **Wisdom:** cultivate depth, loving kindness and inner peace – share your knowledge with others.

I am grateful for all the time I spend with my boomer and senior clients. My life is enhanced by our relationship. And, as my 18-year-old son so eloquently put it the other night on his return from his basketball game with the 45+ "Blues Brothers" from Ste-Agathe, "I love hanging out with old people!"

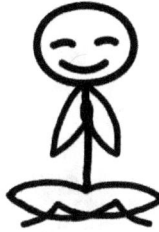

MONTH SIX

Challenge of the Month: MINDFULNESS

Continue with your FTM routine, eat your greens
regularly and practise being mindful

- Mindfulness shifts your thoughts away from your usual preoccupations toward an appreciation of the moment and a larger perspective on life.
- Mindfulness works, in part, by helping you accept your experiences—including painful emotions—rather than reacting to them with aversion and avoidance.
- Mindfulness helps you gain perspective on irrational, maladaptive, and self-defeating thoughts.

WEEK 1
PRACTISE MINDFULNESS

Every thought we have creates our future! This is radical, life-changing information. How do we harness and channel this amazing power? That is this month's challenge: Being Mindful.

Every thought we have is coloured by our conscious and unconscious beliefs and feelings. How can we become aware of this potent yet very subtle reality when our minds are on autopilot, when we are reacting rather than responding? Being mindful is the practise of intentionally focusing our attention on the present moment and accepting whatever thought or feeling is there, without judgement. No good, no bad, just is. When we connect with the present moment and calmly observe our thoughts, feelings and sensations we become more directly aware of them and, by extension, more aware of ourselves. The pace and stress of modern living often leaves us caught up in a stream of thoughts and feelings, trapped in past problems or overwhelmed by future anxieties. With practise, being mindful gives us a sense of mastery over our thoughts and feelings as opposed to being pushed around by them; a victim of our thoughts, so to speak. The goal of being mindful is to achieve a state of alert and focused relaxation by deliberately paying attention to thoughts and sensations without judgement. Non judgement allows our mind to refocus more easily on the present moment. It helps us to focus on what is actually happening rather than on the story we are inventing to try and get approval, to prove ourselves, to defend ourselves or to hide the truth from ourselves and others. (Embarrassing as it sounds, we all do this ...)

So how can we practise being mindful?
- Become more aware of the world around you: notice and watch your thoughts and feelings; wake up to your physical sensations.
- Do one thing at a time. Give it your full attention. Slow down the process and be fully present as it unfolds. Notice what you see, hear, smell, touch and taste. Involve all of your senses and discover the incredible beauty and joy that is available to you (for free!) in the present moment.

- Set a time daily for a more formal mindfulness practise. The techniques include: sitting in a quiet place, doing deep-belly breathing, paying attention to your body, training your mind to observe, focus and filter. You can do this as your first-thing-in-the-morning meditation, after your cup of warm lemon water.

Make a promise to yourself to be vigilant about what you think, say and do. Be aware and mindful of your negative thoughts. You might be surprised how many subversive and self-defeating thoughts you actually have. Where do they come from? What are you protecting? Who are you trying to control? Where are you going with these thoughts? By being mindful we can change our behaviours and attitudes almost effortlessly.

We are creating our lives with our thoughts. What wonderful life are you going to create for yourself? I'll be watching my thoughts. How about you?

WEEK 2
GIVE THE BEST OF YOURSELF

I have been wondering what to write about and it has finally occurred to me: give the best of yourself to everything and everyone.

This thought emerged as a result of the one-week Yoga Teacher Training retreat I did in mid-October. The experience was fabulous; deeply regenerating and transforming. I was struck though on my return - and this surprised me – how much unconscious negativity and aggression was spewing from people's mouths, how much it coloured people's thoughts, and was reflected in their actions. I have to admit that my tender, open, post-retreat heart felt shocked and appalled by it; by the subtle and insidious nature of negativity and how abrasive and painful this experience felt to me, even though it was not directed at me in any way.

Let's define negativity: marked by denial, refusal to accept or approve, not constructive. Negativism: an attitude of skepticism and denial of nearly everything affirmed or suggested by others. Since my return I have had to "harden" myself, without becoming blasé or numb, against the reality of this pervasive, unconscious negative mindset. I would prefer though to live in a gentler, more conscious world. I have made a commitment to myself to be vigilant about what I think, say and do. I hope you will too.

Let's define positive: active and effective in function, to encourage, to support, to be assured and indubitable (I like that one – we need to be indubitable at this point in time). And to make offerings from the heart. I added that one to the definitions I found in the dictionary – they forgot it! :).

The doom and gloom news we are constantly fed and the promotion of fear it cultivates does not help matters. We are being seduced (brainwashed?) into negative thinking, panic and depression. Don't succumb. Listen to yourself talk. Ask yourself: Am I indulging in negativity? Whatever for? What am I getting out of it? Am I trying to distract myself from my own fears, my insecurity or self-doubt? Am I overly perfectionist? Am I bored?

Tips on being positive:

- Be grateful for your life, for all the good and beautiful things in your life, every day.
- Be acutely aware and vigilant about what you think, what you believe, what you say and how you act. If you are being negative, interrupt yourself and reframe.
- Focus on, acknowledge and reward what is good. Offer constructive feedback if necessary, gently and without agenda.
- Become aware of what is good and hopeful. Give your energy and support to it.
- Be sensitive and understanding. Listen. Redirect those who are "stuck in negativity" to simpler things like the blue sky or that beautiful piece of music. If they are still stuck, offer silence.
- ENJOY the moment. Don't sweat the small stuff. Share love (smile, be caring, be helpful, have compassion, take time to be present with one another, don't be afraid to say I love you), release yourself into the delicious, heart-warming, joy-producing, vitalizing light of positive energy.

Today, and every day for the rest of your life, give the best of yourself to everything and everyone. Go on, make a conscious, honest effort to be positive and watch your world, our world transform. Hershey's kisses and bear hugs.

WEEK 3
MAKING PEACE WITH YOUR SOUL

I guess I'll start with making peace with the road construction first! It's been ghastly. Enough said. I take a deep breath in, and on the exhale I focus my attention inward. I empty my mind; still it with one-point focus. I inhale slowly, connect to my center, recharge. I keep my mind still. I exhale slowly and consciously release any tension that I feel. I come back out into the world. The busy, noisy, chaotic, world ... the world of daily dramas, brainwashing media hype and nicely packaged illusions. It's okay. It's my world. How I dance with it is up to me. I choose. The realization that I can choose how I am going to relate to life and its curve balls is immensely empowering. I am not a victim. I have the responsibility for dealing with the consequences of my beliefs, my thoughts, my emotions and my actions. That requires effort. Sometimes it is work. Work I love because it sets me free.

How easily we allow old habits and set patterns to dominate us. Even though they bring us suffering, we accept them with fatalistic resignation, for we are so used to giving in to them. We may idealize freedom, but when it comes to our habits we are often enslaved. Reflection can trigger change, shed light, help us to be a little wiser. And so I bring up the point. If I make peace with the dark feelings and thoughts that are inadvertently provoked by the weather, or anything else for that matter, I am one step closer to making peace with myself. It is a practise. I watch my mind. I am aware of my mind. I take action to redirect my mind towards stillness and peace. If I make peace with myself by being courageous enough to face the truth about myself, I am one step closer to making peace with my soul. It is a practise. Author Sogyal Rinpoche of *The Tibetan Book of Living and Dying* says: "... learning to live is learning to let go. This is the tragedy and the irony of our struggle to hold on: not only is it impossible, but it brings us the very pain we are seeking to avoid. Through weathering change we can learn how to develop a gentle but unshakable composure. Our confidence in ourselves grows, becomes so much greater that goodness and compassion naturally begin to radiate out from us, bringing joy to others."

In Yoga we have the practise of Savasana or, in English, Corpse Pose. One of the practices of Corpse Pose is a short meditation in which you ask yourself whether you are ready to die right now; to leave this Earth in total peace right now! Questions such as "Is there something that I need to say to someone?" or "Is there something I want to do for someone?" or "Is there something I would still like to do?" You will receive an answer intuitively, especially if you are open and listening. Your soul will speak to you. Introspection and contemplation of death will bring you a deeper sense of the meaning of your life and all that you cherish. You will be able to act on this awareness rather than feel regret or remorse because you no longer have the time to. Reflecting on death can bring about a real change in the depths of your heart and wake you up to life.

Making peace with your soul on a daily basis:
1. Breathe and still your mind. Meditation opens you up to the exhilarating spaciousness of your true nature.
2. Practise gratitude and become happier, healthier, and more energetic. Research has shown that gratitude journaling relieves pain and fatigue for people with neuromuscular diseases. Gratitude is actually a gift you give to yourself.
3. Make peace with yourself. Take a good, hard look at everything you have ever done and remind yourself that you have learned.
4. Be kind to yourself. All the self-reproach, guilt, disappointment, self-hatred and anger that you direct at yourself takes you away from peace.
5. Open yourself to love and enrich your life. Step on your pride. Resolve conflict.

It is never too late to start. May peace be with you.

WEEK 4
THE PEACEFUL WARRIOR

Sunday morning I woke up to a White World, pristine, crisp and cold. Beautiful, especially in the sun. I spent all of Sunday afternoon cooking soups, casseroles and muffins for my family, making extra for my son who recently moved out. I listened to the radio - CBC of course - and heard a wonderful show on beauty and how beauty can save the world. Very inspiring. Dan helped peel potatoes and onions. We chatted and giggled and were silent together. Delicious aromas permeated the air and titillated our nostrils. The orange glow of the wood stove kept us warm and cozy. I was happy, contented and relaxed, totally enjoying myself with these simple pleasures. Just living. My spirit was light (maybe even luminous!). I was smiling and surely humming. I was in the flow, surrendering to the moment, moment by moment. I did not allow my mind to distract me with phrases like "I should" or "I have to", or "I want", or with worries, charged emotions or complicated thoughts. I was pure, unadulterated peace and joy! I called my son and left him a message on his cell, "I made food for you." He arrived 25 minutes later. "Are you hungry?" I asked. "Starving." he said. We had dinner and then watched a movie Anthony brought called *Peaceful Warrior* based on a book written by Dan Millman. The movie was about being in the moment, finding peace, beauty and joy, and how to accomplish that. Synchronicity. I love it.

Here are some of the tips shared by those on the path of the Peaceful Warrior:

1. Take out the trash! The trash is anything that is keeping you from the only thing that matters, this moment. Here. Now.

2. If you don't get in the moment, you are going to live your life either in the future or the past.

3. Always keep your mind in the present. By dwelling on the past and regrets of the past, you are not living.

4. When you truly are here and now, you will be amazed at what you can do and how well you can do it.

5. Life is a series of moments. The best we can do is bring more enlightened moments into our lives.

6. The habit is the problem. All you need to do is be conscious about your choices and responsible for your actions.

7. Do regular, moderate exercise. Eat a balanced diet for you. Rest.
8. There are no ordinary moments.
9. There is never nothing going on.
10. Wake up! Live your life. Don't run away from it.
11. You have to decide to get into your heart and be happy.
12. If you look within the heart you will find happiness there, you will find joy there, no matter the circumstances.

So why Peaceful Warrior? Warrior, because we need to be courageous with ourselves in order to cut through illusion and fear. Peaceful, because the answer lies not in fighting or resisting but rather in surrendering. Surrendering to the present moment, surrendering to peace, surrendering to love. To surrender is like making a leap of faith. It means to let go of controlling, to soften the hard shell of defence, to trust your heart and embrace the moment as it is, without judgement. To be a Peaceful Warrior is a life-time of practising. When we appreciate the journey, the beauty of life reveals itself. Happy trails!

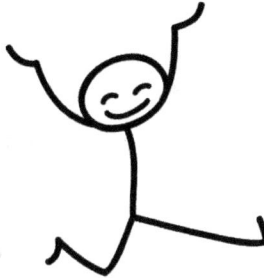

MONTH SEVEN
Challenge of the Month: UP THE ANTE

Up the Ante on your exercise effort and regime

Cardio Protection: Benefits of Improved Aerobic Fitness
1. Improves insulin sensitivity.
2. Helps to manage or prevent Type 2 Diabetes.
3. Preserves bone mineral density.
4. Reduces the risk of coronary artery disease by 50 percent.
5. Helps reduce and maintain the loss of body fat.
6. Lowers the incidence of colon/breast cancer.
7. Lowers elevated blood pressure.
8. Improves balance and prevents falls.
9. Improves cholesterol and triglyceride levels.

WEEK 1
UP THE ANTE!

Did you know that our brains shrink over time? That explains it, some of you are thinking. The average 90-year-old has only half of the wiring they once had. Oh no! The good news? Brains grow. Multi-sensory stimulation, novelty, enriched environments and brainteasers promote neural plasticity by challenging the brain to work in new ways. But here's the kicker: Exercise seems to have the biggest impact on maintaining brain health. If Sudoku is the shovel, exercise is the bulldozer. The hippocampus in particular - the part of the brain responsible for memory - grows most significantly from the challenge of exercise. So if you want to hang onto your marbles, EXERCISE!

Exercise halts brain damage. It regenerates both white and gray matter. It stems cognitive decline! Exercise stimulates all aspects of cognition: improved reasoning, spatial functioning, processing speed, decision-making, learning of balance as well as several kinds of memory. Exercise helps to both eliminate stress as well as renovate the part of the brain that manages stress. Exercise makes us relaxed and happy in a deep and lasting way. It chases away the blues and keeps them away. Exercise bolsters the parts of us that normal aging erodes. It adds life to our years! So here it is from Bruce Grierson's *What Makes Olga Run?*

Aerobic exercise:
- Boosts our central command functions (to think critically and deal with ambiguity).
- Re-insulates the axons of the brain cells, boosts processing speed and creates more reliable connections.
- Has a cognitive multiplier effect – sparks production of neurotransmitters (brain chemicals that relay signals to neurons) and creates more receptors for them in key areas of the brain.
- Turns on genes which keep that positive cycle spinning.

Resistance training:
- Produces brain-building proteins (neurotrophins) which signal brain cells to survive and reproduce.
- Improves executive control – scheduling, planning and dealing with ambiguity.

- Helps pump the heart and simultaneously perform more skillful, more complex movements = superpower boost.
- Combine spatial orientation + variety + explosive heart pump in short blasts = best results.

Sweat equity - intensity and rigour count:
- The hippocampus grows quantitively in relation to intensity.
- Intensity concentrates the physiological benefits of exercise.
- The level of effort is what promotes astounding recovery.
- Ten minutes of high intensity makes you much more fit than 120 minutes of light moving around.
- Intensity is in relation to an individual's activity level and ability - try for 80 percent of your maximum heart rate for short bursts; alternate between intensity and rest (recuperation time).
- There is an intensity threshold where exercise becomes really beneficial - you need to sweat to provoke an adaptation response. Harder is better up to a point. There is a limit. Over-exercising can damage the heart.

Exercise buys us a chance at a long life by lowering the risk of a variety of ailments including heart disease. It reverses the effects of a genetic bad hand (i.e. switches off genes which pre-dispose us to obesity) and promotes the growth of stem cells in muscles. Younger every step of the way! When you add exercise to anything, you get the 'synergy effect'. Exercise makes every good habit more potent. You can introduce exercise at any point, right up into very old age, and reverse decline! So Up the Ante on your exercise effort and regime everyone. That is this month's challenge. Go for it!

WEEK 2
THE IMPORTANCE OF STRENGTH TRAINING

Summer furniture and toys cleaned and put away, check. Garden closed, check. Winter wood delivered and stacked, check. Winter tires installed, check. Outdoor Christmas decorations installed, check. The last geese are long gone. The first snow has come and gone. I am ready for winter. Are you?

For some of us winter restricts our activity. We find ourselves more sedentary, less motivated, less able to go out in the cold weather, snow and ice. There may be other reasons keeping us from regularly making it to our exercise classes, doing outdoor activities or going to the gym. What can we do to counter this and the resulting negative impact on our health?

I would like to suggest that you incorporate strength training into your weekly routine. Strength training can also be done at home. I have observed that too many of us neglect to train our muscles. Why? Perhaps we don't understand the importance of it. We may lack motivation and discipline. Let's face it, strength training is hard work and some of us may be a little lazy. Did you know that from the age of fifty we begin to lose 3 kg of muscle mass every decade ... unless we make the effort to keep our muscles strong.

Here are 9 good reasons for all of us to strength train - no matter our age:

1. Boost brain health and cognitive function.
2. Prevent osteoporosis (or slow the decline) by increasing bone mineral density.
3. Maintain a healthy weight by augmenting muscle mass: strength training is the best way to add lean muscle mass which is an important factor in weight loss.
4. Increase glucose metabolism which means to increase the use of glucose to form energy in the body = more energy
5. Relieve stress, promote deeper sleep - which by the way also promotes weight loss.
6. Improve posture, eliminate back pain and protect against injury.
7. Lower incidence of chronic disease.
8. Maintain autonomy because of greater strength and endur-

ance. The older you are the more vitally important it is to continue strength training.

9. Improve metabolism and psychological well-being.

Here are some important tips to consider when undertaking strength training:

1. Use good technique - get a coach, take a class with a qualified instructor to gain a better understanding of what you are doing, how and why. Start now!

2. Use the right weight - there is no harm in starting gradually. When you can do three sets of 8 repetitions, it's time to go to 10 reps then 12. When you can do that, you can augment the weight. Rest between sets. Don't forget to augment the weight or the level of resistance.

3. Strength train 2 to 3 times a week for a minimum of 30 minutes.

4. Strengthen your core, your back, your arms and your legs.

5. Balance strength training with stretching for best results.

6. Resistance training includes the use of your body weight, free weights, elastics, exercise balls, machines, weighted bars, the Bosu, Kettle bells, VIPR, TRX and the SURGE.

7. Protein builds muscle. Eggs, nuts, legumes (beans) and whole grains are proteins too.

You know what they say "Use it or lose it!" Let's get our heads out of the snow and accept the science that proves that exercise helps to reverse aging. Now you know. If you don't do anything about it you have no one to blame but yourself. Start gradually, every little bit helps to make you feel better. Augment activity as you feel yourself getting stronger. Step by step. Variety improves results. Learn to push harder. Muscle building requires effort. So if you don't have the discipline to do it alone, find a training partner, get a personal trainer or take classes. Your efforts will reward you with many benefits, and enhance your quality of life. Do it now. This is a direct order! Hahaha. I love you, and I know you love me too for reminding you.

WEEK 3
HIGH BLOOD PRESSURE

High blood pressure (HBP) or hypertension affects 1 in 3 Americans and 1 in 5 Canadians. HBP is a major risk factor in heart disease and stroke and can cause problems for the eyes and kidneys. 22 percent of Americans and 17 percent of Canadians affected by HBP are unaware of their condition. Women with HBP have 3 to 5 times greater risk of developing heart disease than women with normal blood pressure. Heart disease and stroke are the leading causes of death in North America. So be aware.

Blood pressure is a measure of the pressure or force of blood against the walls of your arteries. The top number (systolic) represents the pressure when your heart contracts and pushes the blood out. The bottom number (diastolic) represents the lowest pressure when the heart relaxes between beats.

You are considered to have HBP when you get a consistent reading of 140/90 - unless you are diabetic, in which case the reading would be 130/80. Normal blood pressure is 120/80. A reading over 129/84 is considered to be pre-hypertension. Pre-hypertension means you are at risk for developing HBP.

Over time HBP damages blood vessel walls. Scarring promotes the build-up of fatty plaque which narrows and eventually blocks arteries. It also strains the heart and eventually weakens it. Very high blood pressure can cause blood vessels in the brain to burst provoking a stroke. HBP is considered the "silent killer" because you can't see or feel it. Therefore you can't detect symptoms easily. Are you getting scared? Don't be. The good news is that HBP can be easily controlled. Treatments for HBP include both medication and prevention.

Risk Factors that are hard to control:
- **Age** (not again - it's just not fair!).
- **Race** (some races are at greater risk; Afro-Americans, Native Americans, South Asians).
- **Family history** (can be considered due to genetic links).

Risk Factors that are controllable:

- **Blood pressure readings** – take regular readings to stay abreast of the situation.
- **Smoking** – Quit now.
- **Excess alcohol consumption** – enjoy 1 to 2 glasses a night (especially red wine) with a maximum of 9 per week for women and 12 for men.
- **Being overweight** – watch what you eat and drink, watch your portion size, exercise and stay active in order to boost your metabolism, burn calories and replace fat with muscle.
- **Poor diet** – reduce sodium (table salt), cholesterol and processed foods (trans and saturated fats) - read labels! Eat plenty of fresh fruit, leafy green vegetables, nuts and garlic to help regulate blood pressure.
- **Sedentary lifestyle** – participate in an on going exercise program (appropriate to your level of fitness) to strengthen the cardiorespiratory system, increase muscle mass, promote good blood flow, weight loss and the removal of fatty deposits in the blood vessels.
- **Stress** - Learn to manage your stress with conscious breathing, mindfulness and calming meditation. Try stretching, Yoga, Qigong, Tai Chi. Get fresh air. Sleep and rest to rejuvenate your body. Eliminate stressors. Enjoy what you do. Discipline your mind to not indulge in worry and negativity.

HBP medication is the easiest and most reliable means of addressing high or even low BP issues. Can you see now how the four lifestyle habits (hydrate, meditate, move and self-discipline) we integrated in Part 1 - Laying The Foundations - help prevent life-threatening disease? Healthy lifestyle habits help prevent, postpone and even eliminate the need for medication. An ounce of prevention is worth a pound of cure. With proper diagnosis and treatment of HBP you can cut your risk of stroke by 40 percent and heart attacks by up to 25 percent.

If you have been diagnosed with HBP, getting those numbers down is an important part of keeping yourself healthy. Please honour your life, and those who love you and depend on you, by taking care of your health. If you lack discipline and motivation for exercise, join a class. If you haven't got time ... make some! Hugs and kisses.

Please Note:

Ischemic strokes are caused by a blockage of blood flow to the brain (blood clot). Atherosclerosis makes it easier for a clot to form.

Hemorrhagic strokes often result from uncontrolled high blood pressure that causes a weakened artery to burst.

LEARN THE SIGNS OF STROKE

F ACE is it drooping?

A RMS can you raise both

S PEECH is it slurred or jumbled?

T IME to call 9-1-1 rignt away

Act FAST because the quicker you act, the more of the person you save.

© *Heart And Stroke Foundation of Canada, 2014*

---

1. **Face Drooping:** Does one side of the face droop or is it numb? Ask the person to smile.
2. **Arm Weakness:** Is one arm weak or numb? Ask the person to raise both arms. Does one arm drift downward?
3. **Speech Difficulty:** Is speech slurred, is a person unable to speak or hard to understand? Ask the person to repeat a simple sentence, like "the sky is blue." Is the sentence repeated correctly?
4. **Time to Call 9-1-1:** If the person shows any of these symptoms, even if the symptoms go away, call 9-1-1 and get them to the hospital immediately.

For more information and helpful tips go to:
www.heartandstroke.com
www.heartandstroke.ca

WEEK 4
LOVE AND COURAGE

Life throws curve balls. May I share with you? I recently attended a wake for a newborn. Very sad ... so unexpected. Shocking. What to say? What to think? And think we do, to try to comprehend, to explain, to rationalize and maybe, to distance ourselves for a while from feeling. Feeling strong emotions: devastation, sadness, confusion, anger, helplessness, tiredness ... coming and going in waves. Yes, we all know the effort strong emotions demand. The energy they consume, whatever it is that causes them.

The power of love. Oh sweet balm. So much love surrounds the young parents. A big cushion of love, deep, soft and comforting. Family from both sides, and friends, many people to wish little Margot adieu. Not many words because words are quite inadequate in this moment, no theories or concepts, not even promises of a better tomorrow. No. Love and support of family and friends, yes. For strength. For healing. Individual and collective. Because we all need healing in one way or another when we are rudely reminded of the fragility of life. When we are touched by it our heart is opened. And once opened you will feel everything, even what you want to avoid, what you want to forget. To feel strong emotions disturbs, provokes and overwhelms. We need courage to face, to accept and to let go. Only when we hold onto emotions, without letting them resolve do we suffer from them. And then continue to suffer from them. That is the nature of holding on. Accepting and letting go, that is how to dissolve and dissipate emotional intensity. But to do so, you must accept to feel these emotions. Accepting and letting go is a practise. Breathe, accept and let go. Over and over again until the charge is gone. Unconditional love is the key, for it is forgiving and understanding of human frailty. Love is the foundation of emotional courage. If you know love, if you are loved you can heal the heart of all pain. So love. Love yourself, love others, love your world. Be courageous and start to heal yourself, others and this world.

Words of course are easy ... I begin noticing tiredness in myself and also in those around me who are personally concerned. Accepting and letting go needs to be supported by rest. We must allow the energy that is renewing itself to be reinforced by rest. This is true for many situations such as a return to health after illness, recovery from injury, return to understanding after estrangement, burnout, loss, trauma ... everything must be treated tenderly and with care in the beginning so that the return may lead to flowering.

None of us are spared this process, this reality - only in degrees. We must all live it. Go through it whatever it may be. We call it "growth" or "evolution". I pray everyday that my strength not be tested on some impossibly difficult challenge. I try to be conscious, to open my heart, to correct my errors and forgive my trespasses. I accept and let go. I return to the emptiness and fullness of the present moment. Life is a mystery that I wouldn't dare pretend to understand, wouldn't dare pronounce judgement on. Life is for living with all its trials and tribulations, its ups and downs, its joys and sorrows. The heart is worth living for. My little Margot, with your sweetness and beauty, may you rest in peace.

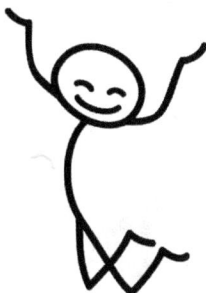

MONTH EIGHT
Challenge of the Month: BALANCE

> Maintaining balance – practise the seven ways
> to spend time every day
> 1. Sleep time   5. Down time
> 2. Physical time   6. Play time
> 3. Focus time   7. Connecting time
> 4. Time in

Balance is dynamic, not static. Balance has to be reestablished continually. Balance is about our bodies in gravity, our physical, emotional or psychological states as well as our mind/body harmony. Balance is connected to what we call centre or being centred. Therefore the closer we stay to center the easier it is to maintain our balance.

Meditation has taught me to be patient, to be still and to let go. Mindfulness has taught me to be aware of what I think and mindful of what I say and do. Yoga, Qigong and other physical practices have taught me focus, breathing and discipline. The arts have taught me pleasure and release. Together they bring me to center. From my center I make better decisions and with more love. Your center is the fulcrum of your balance, the integrating point of all opposites and their tensions, the eye of the storm so to speak, completely still. When we meditate, it is that inner stillness we seek to resonate with - the calm and peaceful stillness that is the even keel of our balance.

WEEK 1
THE ART OF BALANCE

Oh elusive balance! I am a desperate juggling act these days. Time, work, family, work, meal preparation, cleaning, fun, work, rest, writing, new projects, work! How do I manage all the pieces of the puzzle without losing myself? How can I do less when more is begging to be done? I'm losing my precarious hold on balance. This is not how I want to live. Oh elusive balance what can I do?

And because I ask, it comes to me (eventually) in my morning meditation. I relax into the quiet and stillness. Suddenly I can feel it, the source of my tension. An insidious tension contracting the muscles of my forehead and jaw, my neck, shoulders and solar plexus. Slowly choking my life force, leaving me feeling exhausted, burdened, dissatisfied and wondering what happened to joy in my life. And then I get it, the reason. I'm TRYING TOO HARD. Trying to be good. Trying to do it right. Trying to get it off the ground. Trying to make a buck. Trying to be recognized. Trying to get it all done. Trying, trying, trying. Then the light dawns on me. "Trying" comes from fear; the fear of failure ... I won't be good enough. I won't live up to expectations. I'm not doing it the right way. My dream won't come true. Fear, and worrying about the future, create anxiety; a nervous mental state that drains energy and makes living effortful. It's like driving with the handbrake on. Totally useless! You see, no matter whether I try or not, I will have to make that call, write that letter, meet that deadline or clean the house, etc. Trying though involves extra effort: the effort to get your energy moving forward against the resistance created by fear and doubt. What will be will be. If I stay in the present moment I will find a solution – one manageable step at a time, step by constant step. Live the challenges of life with relaxation, clear focus and a positive attitude. STOP TRYING to do it right, to be successful, to get approval, to be loved, to be perfect. Surrender to what is and dare to trust. Go out and get some fresh air. Breathe. Reconnect with yourself and the present moment. Step by step integrate life, health and career in a way that brings you happiness.

Dr. Dan Siegel, a neurobiologist, has some very practical advice for those of us trying to find and maintain balance in this crazy busy world. He proposes seven practical ways to spend your time everyday to optimize brain health, balance and well-being. By giving time and attention daily to these seven essential mental activities, the brain will receive the support it needs to function at its best. Engaging in each of these essential mental activities promotes integration. The brain is better able to coordinate and balance its activities. When we vary our focus of attention we give the brain plenty of opportunities to develop in different ways. This practise reinforces the brain's internal connections, as well as our connections with others and the world around us. There is no set time for each activity. Even a little amount of time spent can produce wonderful results. The key is to engage in all seven areas every day, and that is this Month's challenge!

Seven ways to spend time every day:
- **Sleep time** – When we give the brain the rest it needs, we consolidate learning and recover from the experiences of the day.
- **Physical time** – When we move our bodies we strengthen the brain in many ways.
- **Focus time** – When we closely focus on tasks in a goal-oriented way, we take on challenges that make deep connections in the brain.
- **Time in** – When we direct our attention inward and quietly reflect, focusing on sensations, images, feelings and thoughts, we help to better integrate the different parts of the brain. Meditation, prayer, mindfulness.
- **Down time** – When we are non-focused without any specific goal, and let our minds wander or simply relax, we help the brain recharge.
- **Play time** – When we allow ourselves to be spontaneous or creative, playfully enjoying novel experiences, we help make new connections in the brain.
- **Connecting time** – When we connect with other people (ideally in person), and when we take time to appreciate our connection to the natural world around us, we activate and reinforce the brain's relational circuitry. We make time for those we love.

For everything there is a time and place. Respect and manage your time skillfully each day. Make time work for you rather than against you. Begin your day by paying attention to all 7 areas; then throughout the day make time for each one, however long that might take. You will nurture every aspect of your inner growth and feel fulfilled. Give yourself the gift of time in all areas of your life. You will be blessed with harmony, peace, success and happiness.

If you have been practising with me since the beginning you have all the tools you need to meet the balance challenge. Now practise. Stick to your FTM routine, adjust if necessary, but don't drop it! You will have already completed 2 of the 7 ways! Routine is how we maintain our energy levels, our productivity and happiness. Learn to say no and not feel guilty about it. When you learn to say no, you'll begin to take on only as much as you can handle., leaving yourself room for more downtime and play time. Prioritize. Simplify. Get organized. That's focus time. Delegate if you have to. Find pleasure in whatever it is you are doing. You are learning the art of balance.

WEEK 2
TRAINING FOR FITNESS AND BALANCE

For all of you who walk regularly or do outdoor sports and activities – Bravo! For all of you who take fitness, dance or body/mind classes – Great! For all of you who go to the gym or do regular exercise at home – Way to go! For those of you training for an event such as a race, marathon or sport adventure – Such perseverance! For those of you training as part of your recovery from surgery or illness – five gold stars! Good on you for being motivated, for having discipline and for taking care of yourself. I bet you feel great for it too. You probably have more energy as well as feel a sense of pride and self-satisfaction as a result of your efforts. For those of you who are not with the program yet, it is never too late to start.

Is your fitness training balanced? Are you training in the right way? Are you getting the results you desire? Do you have pain? Ask yourself these questions and answer them intuitively. You will probably find that you know what is missing. People who train for strength, often neglect to stretch (I haven't got the time … I know I should). People who love cardio may neglect to do anything else. People who love to stretch often neglect to do strength training. Extraverted individuals often do not enjoy the more inward journey of Yoga, whereas quieter, calmer people may despise the efforts required for cardio or resistance training. If you have pain you may be tempted to avoid moving, or worse, ignore it and injure yourself more. Each person is different.

Here are some suggestions to reflect on. Include a little of each in your fitness training.

Technique: Good technique requires knowledge and skill. Learn from a qualified teacher, trainer or coach. Investing in acquiring this knowledge can transform your life for the better in many ways.

Posture: Posture is the cornerstone of a successful training program because good posture supports correct biomechanics and ensures core stability and strength. It helps to eliminate pain, prevent injury and wear and tear on the joints. Good posture is efficient and promotes power and speed as a result of improved connection and integration. Good posture reinforces balance and is essential to being centered and agile.

Flexibility: In order to achieve good posture it is important to stretch the many muscles, the fascia and connective tissues which bind the body and limit your range of motion. This stretching needs to be paired with strategic strengthening to be truly effective, especially for older or more tight bodies. Chronically rigid muscles need to be reconditioned with a process which releases, stretches and strengthens the myofascial web (muscle and fascia) to help restore bloodflow and elasticity. This will loosen up your carapace (the armour of your defences) and ensure more effective strength training results. Supple muscles (muscles which can both extend and contract easily) are dynamic, creating a more mobile, agile and graceful body.

Strength training: Strength training is essential for support, stability, power and speed. Strength training also gives us energy, is proven to be good for the brain and helps eliminate pain if we train with proper technique. As we grow older strength keeps us autonomous and allows us to stay active. Being active keeps us strong and engaged in living life to the fullest.

Endurance training: Endurance training is an essential exercise for the heart as well as an anti-depressant. It oxygenates the blood which is good for energy and overall functioning of the body. Alternating between intensity (making the heart work hard) and recuperation (allowing the heart to recover from the effort) trains your heart and vascular system safely as well as provides interesting challenges and variety. Build gradually for best results. Go for fresh air cardio.

Mindfulness/Meditation: New research suggests that mindfulness/meditation can have benefits for health and performance, including improved immune function, lower blood pressure and enhanced cognitive function. More focus. More calm. Better results.

Goals: Setting goals will focus your training objectives and define your needs. Setting realistic goals will improve your rate of success and keep you motivated. You can alter your goals as you improve and discover new areas of strength and weakness. You can set new goals.

Too much, like too little, is not effective. Balance is the key, as is enjoyment, perseverance and good guidance. Balance is the state of being which helps us cope the best with our health needs, with stress and the 'unexpecteds' of life. Balance is an art. Practise and you will improve. I know you can.

WEEK 3
SPINNING THE VITALITY WHEEL

Forward or backward, which way will it go – against the grain or with the flow? The choice is yours. It's up to you. What will YOU do? Making choices sets the vitality wheel in motion. Forward to gain momentum and build vitality with every good choice. Or backward to slip further and further into weakness and decline. Will you choose results or excuses?

Prevention means to avert, to forestall or to effectively stop. Making healthy lifestyle choices is a form of prevention that both protects and enhances your vitality. The three foundational pillars of prevention are cellular nutrition through whole foods, regular physical activity and stress management. Take action in these three areas daily and you are guaranteed to have more energy, feel better and be happier. Sounds easy. And it is, but you have to practise. The more you practise the better you will get at making healthy lifestyle choices. Regular practise leads to good habits. After a while good habits transition into a way of being. Living a healthy lifestyle becomes effortless!

Vitality is your verve, your energy, your life force: strong in body and mind. Stress and your inability to deal with it eat away at your vitality. And stress comes from so many different sources: our diet, our physical environment, our sedentary lifestyles, our relationships, our experiences, our thoughts, our emotions. Stress produces biochemical byproducts: toxins, free radicals, cortisol, which damage the integrity of the cells and alter the body's ability to regenerate itself, to heal itself.

Choice is determination, a decision which sets the life force in motion. Your decision affects the way your energy will move. Not making a choice is a choice, one which will paralyze you and deplete your energy as you struggle with the "push-me-pull-ya" of not doing when you know you should be doing!

Your ability to make good choices is supported by:
1. **Clear Intention** - genuine willingness acts as the catalyst to making change.
2. **Curiosity** – motivates you to acquire knowledge and seek guidance so that you make better choices and achieve greater results.

3. **Discipline** – is the restraint and self-control you must exercise to replace bad habits with good habits.

4. **Patience** – allows you time to change as you learn to commit to your health and well-being - which only gets easier as you become hooked on feeling great!

So here it is plain and simple. To spin your vitality wheel you have to make choices. Good choices will create a positive energy loop which will build in momentum and vitalize your life by providing greater protection against stress, disease and unhappiness. Living a healthy lifestyle daily will provide continued support to the complex biological processes necessary for optimal health. This will build your health and fitness reserve. This will slow down the aging process and speed up your recovery in the case of injury, surgery or illness. If, on the other hand, you neglect to use your will and your discipline to make better choices, stress will begin to chip away at your vitality, eventually overpowering your vitality and leaving you at greater risk for disease, depression and premature aging. Cellular deficiency due to stress, inadequate nutrition and a sedentary lifestyle is cumulative. Prevention is the key to maintaining optimal health, to eliminating pain and to improving quality of life.

We live in a time of worldwide chaos - social, economic, political and individual upheaval. I have observed that many are feeling overwhelmed by what life is dishing out these days and as such are neglecting to care for themselves in the areas of diet, exercise and stress management. A Catch 22! You are distracted, upset, challenged, overwhelmed and therefore you feel you don't have time to exercise, eat right or rest. Ironically it is exactly these things which will help you to better manage and handle the stress that unexpected or uncontrollable events are bringing into your life. If you are neglecting yourself, I invite you to stop a moment and take a deep, quieting breath. Ground yourself and be still so that you can shift the direction of your energy and set your vitality wheel spinning in a life-affirming, forward motion once again. Take control of yourself, your life and your health because if you don't, who will?

WEEK 4
THINK WITH YOUR HEART

Oh my aching heart, my joyful heart, my quivering heart, my outraged heart, my tender heart, my beating heart ... how are you today? Let us look into our hearts, into ourselves, into the truth so that we may become heart stronger, live better and longer.

What is the heart? The heart is so much more than an organ that pumps life-blood throughout the whole organism – although that in itself is so beautiful and magnificent. Those who have heart troubles know what I mean. The rest of us take it for granted. Shame on us.

Have you heard "Think with your heart and feel with your mind." Now what does that mean? Perhaps "feel with your mind" is what Thich Nhat Hanh describes in his book, *The Miracle of Mindfulness*. A state of relaxed, alert receptivity and one-point focus that connects you to the present moment. In this state of mindfulness, we can learn to relate to what is rather than what we imagine and project. As such we can experience what is in the present more keenly, respond with greater calm, be more effective. That is the miracle. Bonnie Bainbridge Cohen, a neuro-developmental therapist and creator of the Body-Mind Centering technique, says that the capacity to be both mindful of the present moment and to be willing to let go and change in the moment is what allows our energy to flow freely, to be continually renewed. Powerful and thought provoking words.

Intuitively I know what "think with your heart" means. Perhaps you do too. In words I would say: thought that is always based on what is right for people, for the earth, for life. A mother often thinks with her heart. The Dalai Lama thinks with his heart. I hope you think with your heart. I had the honour of attending a talk given by Riane Eisler on Building Caring Economics. Very stimulating and interesting. Check out www.globalonenessproject.org for more examples of thinking with your heart.

Each one of us, I believe, has a responsibility to unite heart and mind, that we may break the unwholesome cycle of anxiety, pain and "dis-ease", that we may better celebrate the gift of life. Open your heart to the truth of what is, the way it is. Accept. My friend, Guy, is learning about the hidden gifts of the heart as he delves deeper and deeper into the vast universe of his inner self, despite being faced with the reality of a rare terminal disease. Don't neglect your heart. Take care of that precious organ. Think with your heart and feel with your mind. Be mindful and come into the present moment. Meditate every day and get to know yourself. Learn to handle your emotions and your thoughts. "Your heart is the size of an ocean. Go find yourself in its hidden depths." Rumi

REFLECTION
EVERY DAY IS A NEW BEGINNING

Have you ever thought about how many moments there are in a single day? How much life there is to live right now, if we would just wake up? Lived well, aging empowers you with wisdom, with depth and experience. We learn to be free (hopefully) of the silly traps and lies of marketing, of ego, of false images. My friends, easy living has spoiled us, made our will soft.

Nike says: "Just do it". So do I. Get off the coach, stop complaining, get active. Exercise some discipline with your mind, with your mouth, with your body. Empower yourself by joining a group, consulting an expert, changing your routine, eating better. Be courageous with your fears. Most are pure inventions. Small steps is the painless way . Every day is a new beginning, an opportunity to make a change for the better. I believe in you. Go ahead, believe in yourself.

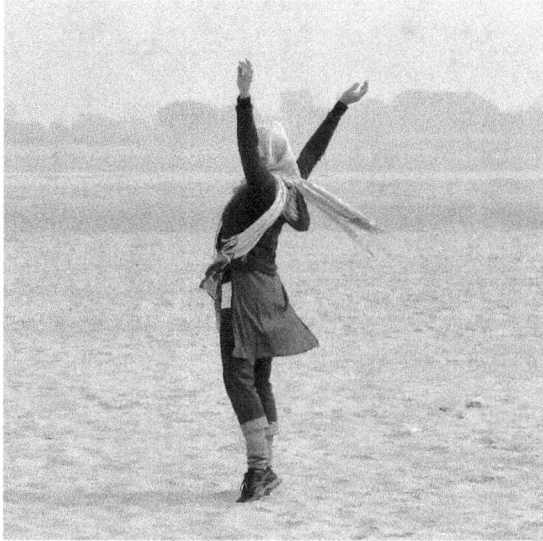

PART THREE
SPREADING YOUR WINGS

"Sometimes your only available transportation
is a leap of faith".

Margaret Shepard

INVITATION
SO, I AM GETTING OLDER!

I have already written about the physiology of aging. I have to admit that I secretly thought that I could beat it! Ha. No such luck despite all my efforts. I am 55 and this year I am really feeling the physical changes. I would be remiss if I neglected to mention all the benefits that I am experiencing as a result of being 55. I am much happier, less dramatic and more at peace. My thinking process is more efficient, unless it requires short-term memory. :) I know what I want and don't want. I fight less. I fool myself a little less. I don't sweat the small stuff. I have more confidence in myself. I have knowledge, expertise, perspective, humility, compassion and understanding. I find that I can be helpful to younger people and to older ones too. I take pleasure in simply being and living. I have come into my own.

Embracing the truth about aging though is not always easy. I find I have to talk to myself, consciously let go of niggly negative feelings. I have to breathe, relax and accept. Over and over again. The pill of acceptance sometimes gets stuck in my throat sideways! My clients chuckle as I share my complaints with them. A knowing and compassionate chuckle ... been there, done that ... just wait. I wish I were 55 again they say.

My friend said she didn't like being in her 50s because that made her so much closer to 60, 70 and 80! "I don't want to get old" said she. We talked about how these fears project us outside of the present moment and cloud the reality of NOW when all is fine, graced by both vitality and maturity. Fears, dislikes and self-criticism fill the body/mind with useless tension, eating away at joy and happiness.

So, be aware of your thoughts! Free yourself from deprecating thoughts, bad feelings and worries about the future. Be responsible and live now. Live well. Honour the gifts of aging. Go deeper. Don't go chasing windmills. Surrender that fight and find grace.

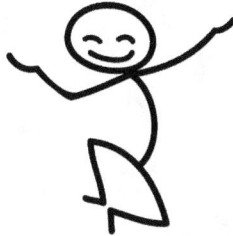

MONTH NINE
Challenge of the Month: CULTIVATE YOUR PASSION

> Choose one new thing to explore for the whole month

A few Suggestions:

1. Visit Museums and attend other cultural events.
2. Take an art class – painting, writing, dancing, music appreciation, pottery.
3. Try a new sport – Kayaking, Dragon Boating, Bicycling, Track and Field, Body Building, Snow Shoeing, Swimming etc.
4. Try new recipes: vegetarian or raw food.
5. Plan a trip and discover a new culture.
6. Learn a new language.

WEEK 1
OH PASSIONATE HEART

Are you "hungry" for life? Or are you just letting it pass you by? Are you "hungry" to taste, to smell, to see, to feel, to touch life in all of its dimensions? Or are you cutting yourself off from discovering that which you do not know, blandly settling for less? Are you "hungry" for new experiences that challenge and stimulate? Or are you content to sit on your laurels, turning a blind eye to the kaleidoscope of possibilities that exist in this great mystery called life? Enthusiasm, excitement, even ardor, are the deeply stirring emotions that compel one to act. Oh passionate heart, dare I awaken you to feel the fire of life and be fearlessly ALIVE? Take a step back. Relax. Open your eyes to behold all that there is and dive in.

Tips to ignite and cultivate passion:

1. **Under-schedule:** leave yourself large swatches of free time.
2. **Engage in unstructured exploration:** expose yourself to many things; go outside your comfort zone. Go on.
3. **Disrupt yourself and your routine:** embrace ambiguity, take risks, be open to controversy and shake things up to gain new perspectives and fresh insights.
4. **Take action:** if something interests you, follow up on it; read, take classes, spend time with others who have the same interest. Watch your interest grow. If you stick with it, your interest may evolve into a life-long passion.
5. **Practise patiently:** actively engage in the step-by-step process of acquiring new skills. Take charge of your mind; focus, nurture and be devoted to the learning process that sustains your passion.
6. **Show interest:** genuine interest leads to meaningful experience. Identify the activity that makes you feel strong and fulfilled, that restores and invigorates you and makes you feel your life is worth living. You are the leader, passion the follower.

Passion is not so much something that you follow, but rather something that you cultivate. Passion is a way of life that embraces curiosity and engagement: pulling up the sleeves, giving thought, care and energy to something that you love, that you believe in, that you want to share. Your passion will inspire passion in others.

Don't give up on being alive. Just start, however awkwardly. Align yourself, leap, soar into the unknown with an open, curious heart and try something new. Persevere. Don't measure results but, rather, your level of enjoyment, personal satisfaction and degree of happiness. That is passion. A vibrant, radiant and sometimes messy life. Go for it. That is this month's challenge: cultivate your passion to feed your soul. Choose one new thing to explore for the whole month. What is it going to be?

One of my passions is travel, another is writing. I send this tip to you from Mexico. Amor y passion.

WEEK 2
DARE I SAY ... LOVE

Last night we celebrated my parents' 50th wedding anniversary. Seventy-five people were invited and almost all came. The evening was perfect. Love was in the air. Cards and gifts of wine, champagne and bouquets of flowers abounded. People were smiling and reconnecting after so many years ... you look just like your mother, is that your son? The last time I saw him ...

On the piano was their wedding album as well as a beautiful slideshow of chronologically arranged photos beginning when they first met in 1954 and continuing right up until the present day. Poignant to say the least. I was touched to witness my parents' evolution; the changes, the similarities, the progression ... so many experiences and memories in fifty years. After dinner we put on Strauss's "Anniversary Waltz" and my Mom came out in her original wedding dress (with a few minor adjustments) and my Dad in a dark suit. They waltzed for us ... "Oh how they danced on the night they were Wed." A truly romantic moment, exquisite I find for this day and age. My Dad made a tender-hearted speech about my Mom and thanked his children for the joy we have given them and for the help putting the party together. A few more speeches followed and even an original blues composition called "50 Years Together" with the back-up "Shuwap" dancers (a family affair). Then the band started up; we danced and the full moon came out to Van Morrison's Moon Dance. Oh boy, what a party.

I share this story with you because I am deeply moved and inspired by love's sovereign power. Love can conquer all: the good, the bad and the hard times. Courage and compassion are love's soldiers, there to help us face the difficulties, to address and overcome them, to help us to grow. For a union to endure one has to dig deep and undertake a journey: the journey of being truthful with oneself and others, of choosing happiness and of setting one's heart free as a result of communication, understanding, acceptance and perseverance. Long-term relationships and family test love ... real love. Sometimes it's not easy or fun. Sometimes it hurts. Oh but the rewards of love, the comfort, safety and joy!

In truth, I do not have a value judgement about marriage, divorce or common law association. They are an essential part of mastering the art of love. I do uphold though the efforts required to discover love and happiness for oneself and, in so doing, for all those around you, whether it be in a personal relationship, in a family or other. I am talking about an inner happiness which radiates like the sun, illuminating both one's self and others.

So let's get to it everyone … for ourselves, our families, our friends and our world. Let the healing begin. Reach for that diamond in the sky with fortitude and faith. Release your pettiness and anger. Stop fighting. Don't allow yourself to be numb. Be humble. Don't be afraid of your tears. Speak your truth with quiet dignity. Listen to and hear what others have to say. Be kind. Be gentle. Forgive.

The efforts made to free the heart yield unexpected results and grace one's life with joy and serenity. This lovely state of being has a profound effect on our health. Research suggests that it is the most important factor affecting our health and well-being – even greater in importance than nutrition and exercise!

Take a deep breath. Make the leap into happiness and boost your health and well being by a thousand fold. Ready? 1, 2, 3, follow me.

WEEK 3
MOVING THROUGH CHANGE

Change. Even when we want it, we hate it! Sometimes we are forced into it. Whatever the reason, change is difficult for most of us. We are wary of the unknown. It makes us feel uncomfortable, insecure. Our confidence in ourselves, our courage, our resolve are tested. What is my new life going to be like? What will I have to give up? What will I gain? All around me I am witness to people going through change. For some it is changes in relationships, in living accommodations or financial situations. For others it is the maddening, frustrating and un-predictable state of their aging bodies. For others yet it is the frighten-ing, heartbreaking reality of the impact disease and/or aging has had on parents or beloved partners, and how that is changing or has changed their lives. Some changes are welcomed. Others, not at all! Change stirs us up, sets the mind to worrying, triggering the stress response which in turn makes everything worse, more complicated! Oh my. Oh painful growth.

Is it possible to adopt an attitude towards change which can ease the process? Yes, I believe so. The first step is to face our resistance to change. Resistance causes tension in the body and conflict in the mind. Resisting consumes a lot of energy because we fight ourselves. We want to control the way things are for fear of what we do not know. We will-fully force and try to shape the situation because we are impatient with the time it takes for us to become familiar with the outcome. Exhaust-ing! More importantly this state of mind inhibits us from experiencing the subtle pleasures which are actually present. Little pleasures which offer us respite and happiness. Some changes are unstoppable. What we have a choice in though is how we live through change.

Tips for easing the hard work of change:
- **Yield** to the fact of change. I don't mean give up but, rather, soften what is rigid and fearful in your perception of your reality. Relax your need to try and control.
- **Accept** the situation. This may require a lot of practise. It is something that comes from opening your heart, courageously feeling the pain without judging it to be good or bad.
- **Let go** of tension, both physically and mentally. This is an action that is initiated by the mind. A mental discipline, a conscious choice of letting go.

- **Come to stillness**. Focusing the mind on the breath to still the body and mind calms the nervous system and allows us to connect to a deeper, more peaceful source of energy which is unemotional and gives us the strength to cope.

Change is moment to moment, awareness to awareness, decision to decision. It is a process which gives us the opportunity to learn about ourselves, to adjust our perceptions and our actions to better fit our new reality. Step by step we begin to recognize and understand what is the truth in the stories we skillfully weave in order to hide from ourselves our feelings of fear, of loss or of inadequacy, of guilt and shame, of anger, and of sadness. This is a trying state of affairs. Arduous really. So yield rather than react, accept rather than resist, let go rather than hold on and come to stillness rather than distress. Practise over and over again. In so doing you will become more tolerant of the intensity. You will transform the ground out of which you are experiencing your life, your change. Many blessings will follow. The more challenging the change, the more support you will require. Love, a helping hand, a receptive ear, expertise ... let us come together with sensitivity and kindness so we may all feel safer and grow stronger in our vulnerability. The light in me honours the light in you.

WEEK 4

In 2013, at 52 years old, I decided to take a four month sabbatical. I needed to rest, reflect, renew. Push the reset button so to speak. My soul was flagging. Freedom Travels is my record of this soul-bolstering, life-changing journey. Enjoy.

FREEDOM TRAVELS PART 1 – BALI

The wind is blowing. The air is soft and warm. The water is a translucent turquoise green. The rhythm of the waves reminds me to let go, let be. I see the rugged terrain of volcano-formed Lombok Island from where I sit on Gili Air Island. I see rain falling over there on the horizon but I can also see the pinks of the setting sun and the silhouette of a twin-masted sailboat. The power of nature once again soothing my over-used nerves. Island life. Hot, sweet, slow. It takes time to unwind. How do I get so wound up?

I am in Indonesia near Bali, halfway around the world! I am travelling with Dan (my partner) and Anthony (my son). Twenty-five hours in a plane. We are on an adventure. And really, it is very different here. Travelling opens your mind to new ideas, new people, unexpected experiences. Adjust, relax, observe. Surrender to the difference. Let yourself be moved, feel uncomfortable even. Embrace the unknown.

Dan is playing the guitar which he bought in Amlapura for $22. A mini adventure which included a 30-minute scooter ride through steep, narrow and winding mountain roads (YEEHAH) and stunning views of rice terraces straight out of National Geographic. Awe inspiring. He is playing with Julien the violin player from France, who studied music in India. Sometimes I sing. What can I say? Life is good and magic happens in an instant, if you allow ...

The snorkeling is absolutely fantastic. Thousands of fish every size, shape and colour from the striped Lion fish to the Pencil fish to the camouflaging Cuttlefish. Spotted turtles too. Big blue starfish in a colourful coral reef teeming with life. Endless expressions and variations on a theme, some so graceful others awkward or quirky looking. Creation was in a most experimental and adventurous phase when designing fish and coral! A whole silent, underwater universe that I can watch like TV, floating effortlessly in the buoyancy of salt water, to the calming sound of my breath ... breathing in and breathing out.

What exactly drew me to Bali I am not sure, but what has struck me, besides the glorious nature, is the culture. Here they practise gratitude for life everyday through the ritual of making offerings. The offerings are both meditation and prayer, prepared by making little baskets from banana leaves and reeds which are filled with flower petals, rice, fruit and other sundries as well as a stick of burning incense, lovingly placed with a blessing. These offerings can be found everywhere: on tables, in front of your door, on the sidewalk, in shrines and at alters. The offerings are made by young and old, male or female and always in a state of deep reverence for the spirit of life. When trees or rocks are wrapped in cloth (and they are even in the remotest of areas) this signifies (and reminds) that these spirits are sacred and must not be harmed in any way.

Making offerings is very serious business but done with such simplicity and sincerity of heart. When you make an offering, you are paying respect, you are honouring, you are caring for, feeling gratitude … quieting the mind, freeing the heart. As such the Balinese are a peaceful and joyful people, giving rather than taking, never aggressive but very persistent if they want to sell you something. They have a day where they pray for the whole world and a day of stillness where everything stops including airplanes. I am humbled by the depth and authenticity of their feeling for the sacredness and magic of life.

They have a lot to learn about garbage though! Plastic, the scourge of all developing nations. It is everywhere, littering the country-side, filling the gullies, floating in the oceans, scarring the beaches. For some reason they just don't see it. They don't seem to realize that the plastic will not decompose and return to the earth like organic matter does. They also don't have the waste management infrastructure to cope with the influx of people. The irony doesn't escape me. They are also suffering the uglification brought on by tourism and the almighty dollar … but who am I to judge their desire for the comforts money can buy?

What is it that I want to share with you with regards to a new beginning? I don't know, try something different? Open your heart and let life live in you. Don't neglect what is sacred. Take care of yourself. Do the smiling meditation often. If now truly is the beginning of an evolution of consciousness as is prophesied, than so be it. What could be better than that in 2013? Do your part and grow in consciousness, in spirit, in love. I am. Let yourself dream my friends. Don't wait to act. Act now!

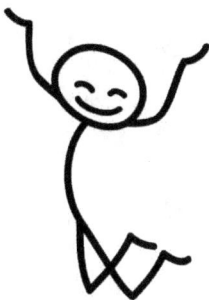

MONTH TEN
Challenge of the Month: EMPOWER YOURSELF

Set an intention you want to commit to, act on and track

"It's been proven that the thoughts we choose have every-thing to do with our emotions. I can tell you that a com-mitment to feeling good can take away a stomach ache, fear, depression, sadness, anxiety — you name it. Any stress signal is a way of alerting you to say the five magic words: I want to feel good. This is your intention to be tranquil and stress free — and it's a way of connecting to spirit".

Wayne Dyer

WEEK 1
CREATE YOUR LIFE

Are you afraid of aging? Evidence indicates that the way we age depends primarily on personal decisions, choices and actions. This means you can exert control over the way you age. But, you have to choose to do so. This is the power that intention holds. Intention is an aim, a purpose, or attitude you commit to. To set an intention is to act to make it happen. Ask yourself, "What do I really want in my life? Health, Love, Happiness, Comfort, Security, Peace, Travel, Adventure, Purpose?" You can have it. Intention is a seed you sow. Align your intention with your authentic desire and empower yourself to create your best life.

Clarity of intent, coupled with mindfulness and awareness, is the most powerful mental creative force you have. For your intent to be realized you must support it with action. The energy and focus you commit to manifesting your intention, combined with perseverance, determine your results.

Tips to setting intentions:

- **Quiet the mind.** The ideal state in which to plant your seed of intention is in the silence of a quiet and peaceful mind, i.e. after meditation, prayer or feelings of gratitude. In nature.

- **Be positive.** Shift your focus from what you don't want to what you DO want. Refrain from using negative words. Yes I can. I want to feel good.

- **Allow your intentions to evolve.** Your feelings and thoughts will become more clear and refined as you evolve in your understanding of what you want. Focus on what your life will look like once your desire has been achieved. Revisit your intentions often but don't hold on to them. Leave room for grace.

- **Track your progress.** Keep track of the actions you take every day towards the realization of your intention. If you want to lose weight, track everything that you eat for 31 days. If you want your financial situation to improve, track every cent you spend for 31 days. If you want to improve your relationship, everyday find something about your partner to be grateful for and tell them. Become aware of yourself so you can consciously align your actions with your intentions.

The classic Vedic text known as the Upanishads declares, "You are what your deepest desire is. As your desire is, so is your intention. As your intention is, so is your will. As your will is, so is your deed. As your deed is, so is your destiny." Set your intention, be clear and take the appropriate action to make it happen.

Overcome the stress of aging by using the power of intention to make your life more satisfying, meaningful and enjoyable. Become the master of your mind. This month's challenge: set an intention you want to commit to, act on and track and, in so doing, empower yourself to live a better, more fulfilling and happy life.

WEEK 2
MIND OVER MATTER

If you have been reading these Tips you know that good health and disease prevention are based on making lifestyle changes in the areas of what you eat, what you do and how you think. In Mindfulness Practise, I talked about how mindfulness, focus and meditation calm and quiet the mind for greater clarity and serenity. In Dare I Say ... Love, I underlined how love and happiness bring joy and beauty into our lives. These powerful emotions are actually manifestations of our thoughts and beliefs.

Scientific research has shown the mind to be so potent that thoughts alone (imagining) about situations, actions, and feelings can produce exactly the same physiological (body) responses as though we were actually doing them! Astounding. The mind is considered to be the most instrumental factor in our health and well-being because the body follows the mind. This statement is not to be taken lightly. But what does it actually mean?

However different thoughts, feelings and actions may seem, they are all expressions of energy. Energy is the animating principle of life. We are energy. Our bodies emit the energy of our thoughts and feelings. The energy we generate with our mind becomes the creative force in our lives. This process is fundamental, a very subtle and complex process resulting in the unique expression that is each one of us. This fact, which we take for granted, is remarkable and magnificent.

I recently watched *The Secret* and was reminded about the law of attraction. Simply stated: whatever you focus your thoughts and feelings on is what you attract. The law of attraction does not discern between good and bad, or right and wrong. The law of attraction matches energy with like energy. This is a profound and provocative thought. Could it be that each and every one of us is totally responsible for our lives, how we live them and what happens in them? Radical. It is much easier to blame others, to find excuses. But, if you allow yourself to consider the idea seriously, a very empowering possibility surfaces. You can consciously create your life.

As a matter of curiosity and conscience, I decided to observe my thoughts and feelings. I was shocked to find how many negative (I use this word to describe what is not affirming) thoughts and feelings I harbour. And I am a positive, upbeat, happy girl! I realized that my negative thoughts whether towards myself, my child, my partner, etc., actually belied feelings of fear: fear of failure, fear of inadequacy, fear of hurt. In truth I was projecting those negative thoughts to protect myself from feeling my fears. Oh so very human ... but not very empowering.

I invite you to observe your thoughts and feelings and replace your "negativity" with triumphant thought, with feelings of gratitude and happiness. Your life will be transformed.

The body follows the mind, and the mind follows the body. They work together in a most beautiful and complex way. La vie est belle!

WEEK 3
MY SELF, MY REFUGE

The melodious honking of the Canada geese and the glorious colours announce that shorter and colder days are on their way. Already?! September was fantastic. The Quebec we all adore. Let's hope that October holds more of the same so we can continue to stock up on vitamin D and cheerfulness. Have you noticed that life is just more wonderful when you are feeling cheerful? Food tastes better, people are nicer and obstacles are easier to overcome. In ideal times cheerfulness is easier to achieve and maintain. Ideal times come and go. We cannot boast that our Planet Earth is in an ideal time. That being so we need to learn how to cultivate and safeguard that ideal condition within ourselves. So where do we turn?

Spiritual teachings of all kinds advance the idea that we are ONE. Science as well searches for common denominators and unifying principles. Life is a supremely vast and complex reality that spirituality, science and we, the individual, seek to grasp and understand. We have the universe (multiple universes). We have the planet (planets). We have life forms (animal, vegetable, human, unknown). We have species and races. We have worlds, continents, countries, communities and families. We have the individual. We have DNA. We have nuclear medicine, particle theory and quantum physics. Matter and Energy. Macrocosm and microcosm, the part reflected in the whole, the whole reflected in the part, visible and invisible. The complexity is astronomical. A mystery's mystery! We do not fully understand the power of our very being. The power to be, to change, to do, to become, to heal, to be at peace, to be part of the whole. Now take a deep breath (after that big brain stretch) and come back to center.

Tibetan Buddhists say that you have to be aware of your death, face it, and prepare for it to fully appreciate life. Not to take it for granted. Not to waste the opportunity for joy, for love, for appreciating beauty and for liberation. Now take a deep breath into your heart center and realize your heart's desire for this precious life.

Vibrating in every part of our organism, our mind, our heart, our cells is this ability to resonate with the whole; the planet, humanity, the universe, the unknown. This truth is so magnificent, so overwhelming that most of us just simply ignore it. And in so doing, we limit ourselves to an unconsciously contracted life, bound by the myriad of stories we tell ourselves (and those fed to us) of unworthiness and powerlessness. Now you may be asking yourself "What drug is Lisa on?" Breathing of course! Please, take a deep breath in and exhale slowly, softly.

I am discovering that breathing is the most direct route to calming myself, to being in the present moment with what really is (nothing and everything), to centering and opening myself so that I can make conscious choices about how I act, rather than react. Breathing slows my life down to a manageable pace by creating space and non-density in my body and mind. Breathing nourishes my cells, improves my circulation, helps eliminate tension and, in so doing, supports my vitality. Breathing in itself is the key to a meditative state of mind. Breathing quiets the nervous system and the voice of ego so that consciousness (your deep intelligence, that which is aware of being part of the whole) can speak clearly to you, guide and direct you in making choices which will help you achieve cheerfulness. So, I say, use all you've got to cultivate cheerfulness and don't neglect the source of unconditional happiness, love and goodness which lies within you. Harmonize your little self and your big self to the melody of the honking Canada geese, to the glorious fall colours, to the deep, quieting and cleansing breath. Lift the corners of your lips and direct your smile inward as you nestle into the center of yourself, refuged in the greatness of ONE.

WEEK 4
FREEDOM TRAVELS PART 2 – BALI

I gaze out onto the vast blue expanse of the Indian Ocean from my seat in Nasa's Warring (local restaurant) on Balangan Beach in south Bali. Wow, what an adventure. In the last six weeks we have walked on white sand beaches, black sand beaches, rock pebble beaches, crushed coral and shell beaches on the east, north, west and south coasts. We have been swimming, snorkeling and surfing. We have hiked through the jungle amongst the Cocoa trees, the Vanilla bean trees, the Bamboo, the Clove, the Papaya, the Mango, the Avocado, the Rambutan and the Banana trees. The rich earthy smell titillating our nostrils. We have felt the charged power of the waterfalls in Les and gleefully rocked, rolled and splashed our way down the Agung, white river rafting. We have played with cheeky monkeys and ridden on the back of elephants. Do you know how a she elephant teases a he elephant? With her trunk of course! And guess where.

It is the rainy season. The warm rain cooling the burning heat of the Bali sun. Swimming in the rain. Laughing in the rain. Riding scooters in the rain. Vroom, vroom up and down the steep, winding mountain roads. Along narrow coastal routes with stunning ocean views. Praying and maneuvering our way through the hazardous, horrendous and smelly traffic of the cities. Off to visit villages, markets, and temples. In Bali, villages specialize in one trade. Villagers make bricks or weave, are woodcarvers or silversmiths. They make kites, are renowned for painting or Batik to name just a few. Their remarkable crafts are acclaimed worldwide. Many are farmers. They cultivate rice, corn, vegetables, ceremonial flowers, fruit, etc. They have chickens, cows, pigs and goats. Everywhere chicks, piglets, kid goats and calves bleat, peep, snort and moo as they chomp, peck and scratch for food along the side of the road. Adorable, but be ready to use your brakes. In Nusa (island) Lembongan their specialty is the cultivation and farming of seaweed. All done by hand. Carrageen, the final product, is used in ice cream to make it smooth and creamy. The average monthly salary is $70.

We attended an elaborate ceremony for protection against evil spirits (always handy) in a huge underground cave in Nusa Penida. We trekked Mt. Rinjani in Lombok, the second highest volcanic mountain in Indonesia at 3700 meters. A three-day, two-night trekking adventure with our wonderful guide, Macho. We camped on the crater rim at 2700m on the thinnest of mats but were warm inside our tent and sleeping bags. Seven hours of trekking a day. The views majestic, the hot springs by the crater lake divine, the sunrises awe-inspiring. Above the clouds, in pristine nature, the stillness is spiritual. I was sore for three days afterwards. Lol. We even partied all night long in wild and crazy Kuta for Anthony's 23rd birthday. Dan and I were the oldest ones there. OMG, LMAO, WTF. Party On! We have met people from Australia, Holland, Germany, Switzerland, and Italy. Russians, Japanese and Swedes, South Africans, Americans and even some Canadians who know people we know! I have met beautiful young people who give me hope for a better world and many over-50 free spirits livin' it up with less. I have been warmly received by the the Balinese people, their children, their families. Treated graciously with kindness and dignity. My heart is full.

I have done the book-reading meditation, the wave-watching meditation, the trekking-Mt. Rinjani meditation, the sitting-and-waiting meditation and, finally, the stillness meditation. I have settled into a peaceful, quiet, worry-free heart and mind. To get there I had to make friends with a host of unsettling feelings and annoying habitual thought patterns. It is easy to say surrender, but for some of us letting go of controlling is a tough, uncomfortable, even scary, process. I had dreams that dredged up old, disturbing feelings. Who knew I had so many. Lol. Many of us avoid stopping and resting for fear of what might arise. How it might hurt us. You can't let go until you face, forgive and accept. In the end, no matter how you cut it, each one of us is fully responsible for ourselves; our thoughts, our feelings, our actions, our choices, our lives. The deeper you go, the more courageous you are; the more loving kindness you have for yourself, the more you let go, the freer you will be, the more peaceful, happy and empowered. It is worth the effort. So let go of wanting to be loved, of needing approval, of trying to please. Let go of worrying what others will think and say. Let go of comparing, of judging, of complaining. Let go of the anger, of vengeful feelings, of worry and sadness. Stop manipulating others and lying to yourself. Open your eyes and see the truly magnificent soul that you are. Take a deep breath and allow yourself to gently release the burden. Let life be what it is and has been. You can do it. I am. Surrender and allow your light to shine.

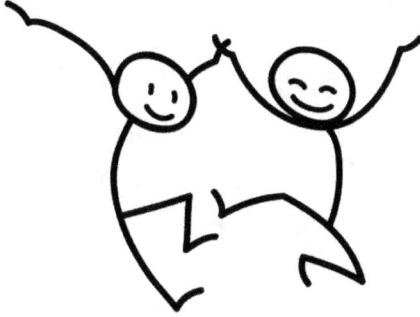

MONTH ELEVEN
Challenge of the Month: INTIMACY

Make time for intimacy and sex

"It is an absolute human certainty that no one can know his own beauty or perceive a sense of his own worth until it has been reflected back to him in the mirror of another loving, caring human being."

John Joseph Powell, *The Secret of Staying in Love*

WEEK 1
MAKE TIME FOR INTIMACY

Let's talk about sex Baby. Let's talk about you and me. Let's talk about all the good things that could be. Let's talk about sex! (Salt-N-Peppa). Midlife does not have to be the end of intimacy. Sexual feelings don't disappear as you age unless you neglect them. The Isis study (a national survey of sexuality and spirituality) found that women in their 60s and 70s were having the best sex of their lives! Communication is key. To maintain a satisfying sex life, talk with your partner. Differences in libidos are common among couples of all ages. Stress, disease, certain medications, being out of shape - all have a negative impact on desire, drive and performance. Although we may want to blame menopause and erectile disfunction, the "sexperts" say this is not entirely right or fair. There are many ways around these issues, but first, you have to want to make the effort. Do you?

The body changes as we age. This is normal. Testosterone levels begin to decline at around 30 by one percent every year. The penis doesn't necessarily react the same way after 50 as it did at 20. Taking longer is normal. Less staying time is normal. Fondling and manual stimulation, it seems, make the critical difference. And how about high heels, a short skirt without panties, a feather boa ... just saying. Menopause affects libido in that the peaks of desire related to ovulation are no longer there. Replace ovulation with the magic of romance guys! Vaginal dryness is common as well. Do what everyone else does, use water-soluble lubricants. And girls, sexy is not a body type but an inner attitude.

Tips for getting in the mood and reviving your sex life:
1. Be mindful of diet, sleep and exercise (sexercise) to help restore libido.
2. Cultivate intimacy: trust, share, talk openly without judgement. You love each other. Even without the fireworks, the erotic flames can burn hot and bright.
3. Take the focus off intercourse by spending more time on foreplay. Slow down, listen to music, drink wine, engage in leisurely whole-body touching, sensual massage, masturbation and oral sex to nourish delightfully erotic and orgasmic "sexperiences".

4. Let go of expectations. Be playful. Open your mind to the unknown. Go on, drop your prudish pretensions and let your hair down. (Mrs. Peacock did it on the kitchen table with the cucumber, or was it Colonel Mustard?)

5. Make changes in your sexual routines; experiment with erotic books or movies, play games and share fantasies, change positions and locations. It works.

6. Focus on the pleasure you can enjoy now rather than on the way it used to be. Many books are available on how to maintain a healthy sex life as you get older.

The physical and energetic bonding which occurs during lovemaking, in whatever form it may take, is profoundly nourishing and satisfying. It transcends the mundane and leaves you grinning and vibrating with the great mystery of life. Alive, present and renewed. This month's challenge: make time for intimacy and sex in your life. Kisses xoxo

WEEK 2
LIVING WITH UNCERTAINTY

Silence. I really need to turn off the radio and the TV ... too much news; bad news, depressing news. Y-gads. The media seem determined to try and convince me – without me becoming aware of it – that I am a powerless victim! God forbid. Fortunately, as a result of being mindful, I am now preventing this insidious, collective-unconscious negativity from taking root in my body and mind. I feel like Joan of Arc with sword and shield – I say NO to mind control!

At the beginning of February I became increasingly aware of an acute state of tension in my clients – such as I have never witnessed before. My antenna went up! Intuitively I felt that I was witnessing an unconscious reaction to the uncertainty of the times we are living in.* I felt and saw a state of tension which reflected back to me a profound state of stress, fear and sense of powerlessness – all unconscious. Powerlessness can lead to despondency, despondency to inaction, inaction to depression ... and around and around in an ever-deepening downward spiral of negativity. I am getting depressed just writing about it! Lol

We addressed this tension by:
- Becoming aware of the tension and by naming the fears;
- Doing relaxation and breathing exercises;
- Cultivating body awareness and control of our bodies;
- Encouraging self-responsibility and empowerment;
- Having fun and experiencing well-being.

It suddenly dawned on me. While the media and powers that be are trying to brainwash me into believing that the "the sky is falling", the actual truth is that my life is good, very good. In that moment of reflection the spiritual teaching of "being in the present moment" struck me as pure brilliance. Ah ha! You never need the present moment more than when times are tough. **Awareness of the present moment** provides you with the opportunity to ground yourself in what is real in your life and to appreciate what you have rather than worry about what you don't have. That simple process of awareness is key to stopping

* *This tip was written a few months following the world economic crisis of 2008.*

the uncertainty, the fear and the negativity from dominating your life. Eckart Tolle writes beautifully about this in his book *The Power of Now*. We must be actively involved with the precious gift of life.

Practical tips for dealing with uncertainty and tension:
1. Be grateful for what you have right now.
2. Breathe consciously and ground yourself in the present moment so you can be aware of what you have.
3. Quiet your mind through meditation, exercise, sports, art, going to the spa, being in nature, listening to music etc.
4. Join a Yoga, Qigong or Tai Chi class to practise breathing and "being in the present moment".
5. Don't allow fear to be your master; empower yourself to enjoy your life right now.

Breathe deeply and slowly. Relax your neck and shoulders. Let your weight drop down into your hands, your seat and your feet. Quiet your mind by focusing on your breath and the body sensation of your feet being in contact with the earth. **Now you are in the present moment.** Open your eyes and look around to see what is real right now. Appreciate what you have, appreciate the beautiful day, or the innocence of a young child, or the playfulness of your beloved pet or the setting sun … there may be no end to what you can appreciate and be grateful for, if you just start and try. Namaste.

WEEK 3
SUCCESSFUL AGING IS ACTIVE AGING

A ten-year study on Aging by the MacArthur Foundation found that individual choices and behaviours, attained through individual choice and effort, determine how people age to a much greater extent than previously thought. The study contrasted usual aging with successful aging. Usual aging describes the elderly who are functioning well, yet are at substantial risk for disease and disability. Successful aging is the ability to maintain low risk of disease and disease-related disability, high mental and physical functioning and an active engagement in life. The study concludes that individuals can have a dramatic impact on their own success or failure in aging. Take note my friends. It's up to you!

So what is the secret to living longer and aging better? According to the Journal on Active Aging*:

1. Each individual must take personal responsibility for his/her health and welfare as a way to decrease the risks of developing disease.
2. Lifestyle choices play a huge role in whether or not we develop major diseases.
3. Most experts now acknowledge that at least half of all people die early because of illness caused by lifestyle choices, dietary factors and behavioural patterns.
4. Every day people risk their future by what they do not do. It is never too late to start! Lower the risk for premature death and disability by taking action now.

Self Responsibility
Older adults flourish when they maintain the highest possible physical and mental function. Successful agers work on maintaining physical and mental function. They identify risk and work with available medical knowledge, natural alternatives and technology to change the future. Successful agers are not fatalistic about the setbacks of aging. They actively intervene to change the course of what was previously considered inevitable. They don't quit; they adapt. They have a more youthful view and believe in their ability to learn, grow and to stay in the mainstream of life. Take responsibility for your health and well being by making good lifestyle choices.

Physical Activity

With regard to physical activity, few things have a more profound effect on bodily functions than exercise. When you exercise every system revs up: metabolic, biochemical, hormonal, temperature regulation, function, cardiovascular respiration. Epidemiological studies show that active older adults are less likely to experience a decline in function with age, and that physical activity improves their function as well as reduces the risk of dementia and cognitive decline. "Use it or lose it" as the saying goes. Choose active living and participate in your own healthcare and successful aging.

Attitude and Engagement

Social involvement has been determined to be the most powerful predictor of healthy aging. Attitude matters. Pessimists die on average eight years younger than people with a positive outlook on life. Human beings were blueprinted for joy and fun ... we won't live forever, but we can't live like there is no tomorrow, because tomorrow is coming. According to the ICAA (International Council on Active Aging) the key to encouraging older adults to remain active and adopt healthier lifestyles is engagement – a pursuit that is engaging and meaningful to the individual. When engaged an individual is focused on the experience and finds value in the activity. People who are engaged are healthier and are less likely to spiral downward into isolation and depression. There are many ways to become more engaged in your life, your family's life and in the community.

Here are some suggestions:
1. **You are never too old to learn!** Re-examine your interests, your passions and your desires. Choose something and follow through with it whether it be taking a painting, writing or dance class; a cooking, computer, or woodworking class, or any class for that matter. Local community centers offer a wide range of possibilities. Discover and learn something new.
2. **Share your knowledge.** Teach your skills to a younger person, i.e. knitting, sewing, cooking, mechanics, gardening, kite flying, reading, etc. If you love it someone out there will love it too. The exchange is enriching and meaningful for both of you.
3. **Volunteer.** Volunteers are a vital and essential component of community life, and will be for years to come. Volunteering is

action with higher purpose and, as such, benefits both heart and mind. Let's help prepare the way by encouraging children of all ages to help our senior citizens.

4. **Mentor.** I have had the benefit of a few mentors in my life, and their input has been invaluable to my success and happiness. If someone asks you to help them, consider it. A mentor doesn't do the work. He or she guides that work.

5. **Initiate or support a project.** Help improve your community. Make contributions by participating on committees, by sharing your expertise, by networking with business partners, by sharing your resources.

6. **Care.** Care to listen. Care to act. Care to be involved. Care to help. Your contributions are vital to the growth and success of the community, as well as being meaningful and vital to you.

We often underestimate ourselves. Little gestures are just as significant as large ones. Little gestures are intimate. They provide a one-on-one opportunity to touch the heart in ways that heal. A kind word, a helping hand and understanding soothe the soul. My soul has been soothed in so many ways, and my spirit brightened, by the caring exchanges I have had with my senior and boomer clients. So too for you. Come on everyone, put your ego and your worries aside. Let's actively participate in our lives and create a better, more wholesome world. Yes we can.

* Journal on Active Aging Magazine - September October 2012

WEEK 4
FREEDOM TRAVELS PART 3 - UNION ISLAND, CARIBBEAN

After six weeks of leisure it is time for centering, a necessary and important step in the process of personal transformation. For those of you who may not know, I am on a four-month sabbatical. My gift to myself for my 53rd birthday. I felt the need to stop. To rest. To reflect on my life. The last twenty years have gone by so fast. Can you imagine the next twenty? I don't have a moment to waste being unhappy, in denial or in limbo. Do you?

Dan and Anthony have returned home. I am now alone and it is a healing balm. As wives and mothers we often put the needs and happiness of others before our own. This is neither good nor bad. Call it maternal instinct. Alone time though is essential to centering. Don't call this selfish, but rather connection with self. No one can do it for me or for you.

I choose two weeks of Yoga and raw food. I rent a bicycle with a basket, register at the Radiantly Alive Yoga Studio and locate all the raw food joints in Ubud. I am on a mission! Two Yoga classes a day for 10 days. Green juices, a variety of fresh raw food dishes 3 times a day, the occasional 12$ massage, facial and pedicure and some live entertainment in the evening. I am in heaven. My body feels fantastic. My heart and mind are calm and peaceful. I am radiantly alive, cleansed and centered.

February 16th, 9:55 departure from Montreal to Barbados. Believe it or not I am off again. This time it is with my three brothers to visit my Mom and Dad for a week in the Caribbean – a very generous gift from them. A nuclear family reunion. This should be interesting. Imagine being picked up by boat in the dark by your parents, both over 75. How cool is that? Night boating from Canouan to Union Island. Hug, hug, kiss, kiss, big smiles, 'tit Ponche and beer. We are lucky. The weather is perfect. Moonlight, stars and smooth sailing. As I listen to the excited chatter I become mesmerized by the beauty of the moonlight reflecting on the water, by the stars and the silvery blue hue everything is bathed in. My heart is bursting with gratitude. I pinch myself. Is this for real?

Family dynamics run deep, generations deep. Irritations and confrontations are almost inevitable. Learning to move with them, grow from them and heal from them is a challenge but also an opportunity to choose love, practise honesty with self and cultivate compassion. The Chinese Book of Changes, *The I Ching* refers to the family unit as the blueprint for life in society. The love of family is there to help us overcome the traps of ego, to develop patience by being persevering, accepting and forgiving and to activate one's sense of fraternity and solidarity. To reach the dream of a peaceful, fair world we must start in our own homes. I feel very fortunate that I come from a loving family. We can pull together under any circumstance, weather our differences and misunderstandings in order to secure the whole. This is not true of all families. Sometimes the dynamics are extremely complicated, unhealthy and hurtful. I invite everyone though to do their best to accept the truth of their family dynamics, forgive and face the challenge in the best way that they can. Remember, the effort you make will release your heart from anger, from sadness, from fear and set you free.

In my travels I have encountered so many people of all ages, from all over the world, each one with a unique life and story. Conclusion? There are numerous ways to dream, create and live your life. As my mind opens, preconceptions and judgements dissolve. Most of the people I have met are not wealthy, including myself. They are resourceful and enterprising. They are passionate and organized. They do not fear the unknown but rather revel in finding solutions. What kind of life are you going to create for yourself? This is the question I will be reflecting on as I head out to San Miguel de Allende, Mexico for the last leg of my trip. Y tu?

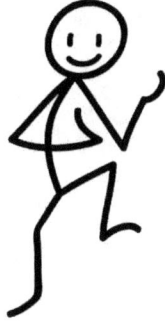

MONTH TWELVE
Challenge of the Month: JOYFULLY ALIVE

Experience simple pleasures that fill you with Joy

Laughter is excellent medicine. Did you know that laughter can:
- lower blood pressure
- increase circulation
- be a fun workout for your abdominal muscles
- reduce stress hormones such as cortisol and adrenaline
- increase the response of disease-killing cells
- defend against respiratory infections - even the common cold
- increase memory and learning
- improve alertness and creativity

Tell me, what is the difference between snowmen and snowladies?
Snowballs.

WEEK 1
DANCE WITH LIFE

The honour and privilege of life is to live it. I hope you are living yours to the fullest, enjoying the richness and beauty that is vibrating right in front of your nose. The beauty of a magnificent blue sky or the melodious gift of bird song or the purr of a contented cat. Simple pleasures can fill you up with joy. You just have to be present enough to appreciate them. If you are spending your time complaining ... Stop. If your words are negative ... Be Silent. If your thoughts are heavy and glum ... Feel Gratitude for Something. Choose to dance with life rather than fight with it. This month's challenge is practising simple pleasures that fill you with Joy!

The concept of self-responsibility is not sufficiently valued in our culture. But there you have it, whether you like it or not, your actions, your thoughts and your words are determining factors in your life. They actually create your life. I invite everyone to embrace more fully the notion of self-responsibility. I encourage everyone to take the necessary steps and actions required to improve their health and quality of life – in those ways that you can. Be aware of your actions, thoughts and feelings and how they affect you and others. Right the wrongs. Be courageous. Be honest with yourself. We are not perfect. We are human. People so often say "It's hard." No, it is not hard; fighting yourself is hard. Feeling angry and miserable is hard. Being unhappy is hard. Taking care of yourself and your needs is to give love to yourself. Come on, you deserve it.

Life is challenging. We suffer hardships: the hardships of youth, the hardships of middle age, the hardships of aging. Hardship is part of life, of learning and growing. We cannot seriously expect not to have any! The key lies not in denying hardship but, rather, in HOW we handle hardship. I know I sound like a broken record, but what we think, what we believe, what we fear and how we act transform experience. Surely, there is someone on the planet who is suffering as much, or perhaps more, than you. Slow down. Calm yourself. Open yourself to the spiritual dimension of being and "see the light" so to speak. Celebrate the lightness of being rather than the darkness of being. This being said, let me also acknowledge that some challenges are particularly devastating or painful. Grieving takes time. Healing takes time. I honour you and your courage.

I have been young, foolish, dramatic, confused and angry. I am no longer (or at least not most of the time). However I would not trade the peace of mind I have acquired to be 20 again ... although I might like to stay 50 for another 10 years. I feel so alive when I share joy, love and understanding. We help each other and create meaningful experiences when we exchange knowledge, kindness and truth. We all have so much to give to each other. Important individual and social needs can be met through simple joy-filled exchanges. Won't you join in this beautiful dance?

WEEK 2
THE RUSH IS ON!

Christmas is right around the corner. The pressure is mounting! The rush is on. Christmas stress is here!

I have good news about stress. Close your mouth and read on. Recent studies reveal that if you believe stress is healthy for you, your body believes it and makes your response to stress healthier! When you change your mind about stress, you can change your body's response to it. That is what science now proves. For example rather than have your blood vessels constrict when you feel stress (which over the long term is very hard on the heart muscle), the vessels remain dilated. Stress is bad for you only if you believe it to be! Revolutionary thinking my friends.

The stress response is a preparedness tool; it is not the enemy. We can turn stress into a performance booster by the way we think about it. It's there to make us work better under duress. It heightens our senses, steels our nerves and increases our attention to detail. We need it. We can learn to reappraise the stress response. We can reduce, sidestep, or repurpose the actual physiological changes to transform negative effects into positive and healthy ones. Wow!

Here's another very interesting fact about stress and the inherent genius of the miracle we are. Our stress response has a built-in mechanism for stress resilience. It's called Oxytocin. Oxytocin is a neurohormone which is secreted equally to Adrenaline (which is what makes our hearts race during the stress response). Oxytocin fine-tunes our brain's social instincts. It moves us to strengthen close relationships, to crave physical contact with friends and family - that is why it is called the cuddle hormone (it is also secreted during breast feeding). Oxytocin increases our sense of compassion which, in turn, inspires us to become more open, more willing to help and support the people we care about. Our hearts have receptors for Oxytocin. Oxytocin helps our heart cells to regenerate and heal from stress-induced damage! Fantastic no? It's a natural anti-inflammatory and helps to keep the blood vessels relaxed and dilated. Oxytocin strengthens our hearts. All of these benefits are enhanced by social contact and social support (reaching out, giving and receiving, hugging). When you seek support or help someone else you release more Oxytocin. Your stress response becomes healthier, and you recover faster from stress. You get better at stress. To know more look up Kelly McGonigal's TED Talk. Human connection, through the heart, literally heals us. A beautiful design.

Practical tips for a joyful holiday season:

1. Practise gratitude, acceptance and forgiveness - which is the same as practising love.
2. Keep in mind that there is beauty in simplicity, grace in expressing heartfelt feelings and blessings in remembering those less fortunate.
3. Acknowledge those who are working hard to prepare meals and organize family celebrations.
4. Be grateful for their efforts and understanding of their stress. Give a kind word of praise and lend a helping hand.
5. Ask for help when you need it.
6. God is perfect but not us! So relax. Have a little faith and let it be.
7. Be mindful and respectful. Alcohol abuse is quite common during the holidays and often leads to ugliness and aggressive behaviour. Don't ruin the family gathering. Drink a glass of water for every alcoholic beverage.
8. Learn to live with differences. Try not to take things personally. Allow the other person their beliefs. They don't have to become yours. There is room for both. Agree to disagree.
9. Breathe slowly, return to your center if your emotions, or anybody else's for that matter, are getting out of hand.
10. If you are sick it is better to stay home. You wouldn't want to make everyone else sick!
11. Get lots of fresh air.
12. And finally, keep the stuffing for the turkey. :)

Face your stress my friends. Discipline your mind and find the courage to change the habits which cause you to suffer your stress. Make the leap and embrace this opportunity to transform Christmas stress into a celebration of the true meaning of Christmas. Meet the challenge. Give from the heart and come together with family and friends in love and joy. Merry Christmas and Happy New Year to you all. I am off to India to transform my stress into a joyful adventure. Blessssssings.

WEEK 3
GRATITUDE

Gratitude is an extraordinary energy that brings inner satisfaction and an immeasurable sense of self-esteem. We often feel obliged to be grateful towards others or towards external situations, but we forget to be thankful towards ourselves for the actions taken and the efforts made in our own growth. To have gratitude for ourselves is a way to acknowledge ourselves, recognize our values and cultivate dignity.

The feelings of love and kindness, which the energy of gratitude engenders, permit us to continue on our evolutionary path with courage and pride. The fact that we recognize ourselves for what we are allows us to be gentle, compassionate and accepting of our weaknesses as we grow along this path. Gratitude allows us to feel harmony and, as such, removes us from the sadness, intolerance, inflexibility and harshness with which we often judge ourselves and others.

Gratitude is inner peace and serenity. When we take the time to practise gratitude, acceptance and loving kindness toward ourselves we make room in our hearts for forgiveness. We can then forgive ourselves and others. This inner state of lightness and well-being, or inner renewal, alters our perceptions. And, almost as by magic, it alters how we are perceived and changes the overall dynamic of our lives. And, it is so good.

To feel gratitude in your heart sets a vibration in motion that promotes balanced health. Gratitude dissolves stress, anxiety and the need for performance, quiets the mind and relaxes the entire nervous system. When we can process our feelings and our thoughts with feelings of gratitude, the power of love radiates outward from us into our environment, becoming a source of well-being and lightness for all those around us. The light in me honours the light in you.

WEEK 4
FREEDOM TRAVELS PART 4 - SAN MIGUEL DE ALLENDE, MEXICO

I absorb glorious Mexico into every one of my cells as I scan the horizon of San Miguel de Allende from the rooftop of my apartment. I can see the Paróquia (parish church), its multiple pink spires all lit up against the indigo night sky as well as three other beautiful church domes. Everything is twinkling. I lift my eyes to the sky, to the stars and then back down to the warm lights of this elegant 18th century colonial city. My amazing four-month sabbatical is nearly over. My journey has been rich and varied. I have had the opportunity to rest deeply, to release many layers of accumulated tension, to be still and worry-free, to meet myself in a new way. I am invigorated by it, opened and softened. My heart and all my feelings are grounded in the present moment. My mind is clear. My intuition is razor sharp, my ability to follow it at optimum level. My spirit is free because I have given myself the permission to let go of all the images running my life such as being a mother, being a wife, being the provider, being a business owner. This experiment has taught me to be aware of the many choices I make based on the image of being rather than my true feeling. And, more importantly, how habitual and unconscious those thoughts and actions are, and how they keep me from truth. Truth with myself has made me happier, less manipulative, less neurotic and confused, more balanced. I have empowered myself in the kindest and gentlest of ways to be wholly myself.

Occasionally on this trip, I have been confronted by the stress, the harshness, the ugliness of a world disconnected from the heart, driven by greed, distorted belief systems and unenlightened business practises. I take a deep breath, root into the earth for strength, straighten my spine and try to inject a little light, a little love and understanding into the confusion, the hurt, the numbness. The effort does not leave me unscathed. I have to work at regaining my serenity. The work makes me stronger. Buddhists say life is suffering. They do not exaggerate. But these days my rebound is spritely, full of acceptance, relaxation and optimism. What can I do other than my best? Peel back the layers of the onion, strip myself of pretension, ambition, desire, stand there naked and raw, delicately perched on the instability of my balance, breathing deeply, taking it all in?

Mexico is very different from Bali. There is a wildness here, a fire in the heart, a dry starkness to the land. Powerful, magical even, I would say. An underbelly rife with the dark passions of pride, of pain, of thirst for blood. Beware of what you wish for. My passions are stirred. I am breaking the mold, stepping out into unchartered ground, daring to let go of my image of myself, of that rigorous self-control that I have exercised my whole life. This is not without danger but is also very stimulating and enlivening. Fortunately, I have not yet danced on the top of the bar. I have kept my clothes on and despite bar hopping until 5am did not disgrace myself by falling over or vomiting in the street. Lol. Not even close. But I danced and laughed 20 years off my life. Let it be. Balance is more challenging when passions are afire and sensual pleasures indulged. Fortunately my discipline and lifestyle habits help me to stay healthy and, even more importantly, to return to center. Passion is not the right guide though. Breath is. Center is. A quiet mind is. Passion is the spice. Center is the way. Let me weave a glorious life tapestry with both!

Mexico vibrates with a sense of community, with the love and strength which comes from family values. We hug and laugh and help each other. The time I spend with younger people is connecting me to the vibrant pulse of change and evolution. Their vitality, their ideas, their desires and ways are energizing me, waking me up. In return I share with them my wisdom, my experience, my patience and love. Let us not forget the importance of intergenerational exchange. Let us not push each other away.

I have met so many people here but a few have really touched my heart. Gentleman Steve - a retired lawyer from Boston who lives in gratitude for all that life has given him and who has a daily practise of doing acts of kindness. Wonderful Aprylle – a gracious and luminous young woman from England open to the unknown, skilled in meeting people and making things happen. Quirky Daniel – the young and very smart Mexican boy, searching for his identity with great humour and heart. Earthy Rosa - the quintessential Mexican mama, lively, round, generous and full of joy. Wandering Minstrel Mark – the artist from the "cities of the world", rich in experience and stories, searching for balance and release. Visceral Lucia – the amazing powerhouse young woman from Bologna who speaks truth with such insight, humour and passion, and Spacious Tim – the Tango-dancing psychologist from Vancouver, filled with compassion for the fragile human psyche and the journey.

I am grateful to all of these people who have graced my life with their beauty, their fragility, their courage on a quest for a better, more true life. We are all so different, brought together by our desire to experience more than spoon-fed illusions, corporate lies or denial of truth. We hunger to feel, taste, hear, smell, touch life. Vibrate, express, exchange and love. I feel so alive.

I invite all of us to step out of our comfort zone and leap into the unknown with courage and love for ourselves, shake up what has become staid and stodgy and bite into life with vigour and passion. I am and so can you. Breathe, ground yourself and let your heart lead the way.

REFLECTION
CAN I SAY YES TO LIFE?

I hope you are taking the time to enjoy yourself. Don't take for granted the small gifts like the fanciful firefly or the bigger gifts of the challenges which make you grow. Please don't take for granted those who love and care for you the most. Open your eyes and see beauty. Open your ears and hear beauty. Open your heart and feel love. Open your arms and receive the gift of being alive.

The choice is yours. This fact is so very important to accept, to understand, to embrace. No matter what life is like for you at this moment – and we know that for some it is easy, for others it is not and for others still it is extremely difficult - how you experience it, remains your choice. How you deal with your challenges is your personal journey. Challenges help us cultivate self-responsibility. They challenge our motivation, our determination, our perseverance. They help build our resilience. Most of us are still working hard on mastering the skill of mental discipline and of surrendering to what is ... and so continues the roller coaster lessons of life, as we slowly evolve in consciousness, in ability, in happiness.

I invite you to be full of courage. Catch yourself when you are thinking, speaking or acting in a way which is deprecating, non-constructive, mean, rude or full of complaint and self-pity. Can you say YES to life? YES to health and the corresponding effort of will. YES to yourself; forgiving, gentle and kind. Can you choose to let go of your resistance to the way things are? If you can't, for whatever reason, then say YES to as many things as you can. When you say YES you allow your vital energy to flow, to grow stronger and become more powerful; to move you onward in the most satisfying of ways. Cultivate this important dialogue with yourself. Take an honest look. You have everything to gain. Continue to make good daily lifestyle choices in the area of nutrition, physical activity and stress management. Watch your attitude towards life. Start anew everyday. Feel good, enjoy, share, relax deeply and fortify yourself. Take a deep, cleansing breath, and on the exhale sigh a soft haaaaaa of pleasure. Lift the corner of your lips and do the smiling meditation. Feel it in your heart and welcome that little seed of joy which is sprouting, growing and blooming as you nurture and nourish it with a YES to life.

CONCLUSION
HOW DID YOU DO?

One year ago I started the "For One Month" challenge with you. Every month I offered a simple tip, in the areas of nutrition, mind management and physical activity for you to practise on a daily basis, the idea being that a daily practise would allow you to observe the benefits your actions have had on how you feel, look, think and act. In short, regular practise develops good habits, and good habits over time evolve into a way of life. That which was difficult, or may even have seemed impossible in the beginning has become natural. Good habits are the foundation of good health. Good health is your key to feeling great, to being happy and to living the life you desire.

The time has come to bring this challenge to an end. Here is a recap of the challenges. Check off the ones you tried. Mark with an X the ones which have become good habits. Did you learn anything about yourself? What?

1. **Hydrate:** drink a glass of warm water wixed with the juice of half a lemon first thing every morning.
2. **Meditation:** take 5 – 10 minutes to sit quietly and still your mind before you start your busy day.
3. **Get Moving:** 15-20 minutes every morning. Get fresh air (walk the dog, walk yourself, do Yoga, Qigong or your back exercises).
4. **Discipline:** practise being disciplined by committing 100 percent and choosing attainable objectives - like the ones above!
5. **Eat Your Greens:** incorporate them into your meals, smoothies or juices. Eat a rainbow of coloured food to get a maximum of vitamins, phytonutrients, enzymes and minerals.
6. **Mindfulness:** become aware of your thoughts, your words, feelings and actions. Reframe to allow more positive and more empowered thoughts and free your spirit.
7. **Up The Ante:** increase the intensity of your physical activity. Include weights, pushing harder and sweating.
8. **Balance:** practise finding and maintaining your balance - body and mind.

9. **Cultivate Your Passion:** open your heart and mind to the new, the different, the unknown. Practise diligently and with pleasure to acquire skills and sustain your passion.

10. **Empower Yourself:** set an intention you want to commit to, act on and track to create the life you desire.

11. **Intimacy:** make time for intimacy and sex with the one you love. Shake it up and ignite the fire and your life.

12. **Joyfully Alive:** practise simple pleasures that fill you with Joy. Dance with life rather than fight with it and transform your stress into a positive force.

A "first-thing-in-the-morning" or FTM routine, although not always easy to keep because of busy schedules, has a profoundly positive effect on the outcome of my day, day after day. Eating my greens and juicing has given me a boost of energy, has improved my digestive health and has led to radiant skin. Being mindful has helped me to better manage my thoughts and emotions which has led to greater peace and happiness. Upping the ante on physical activity is the best way to both renovate the brain and promote optimal functioning. Passion makes life richer and more interesting. Sharing intimacy has allowed me to grow deeper in my understanding of love in a long-term relationship and flower, as a result of the support and comfort which comes from honesty and trusting someone implicitly. Setting intentions and staying engaged in your life are so important to finding fulfillment and to aging successfully. Discipline and balance are the guardians of the practice of being responsible for yourself, your health and your happiness - a practice which leads to joy and joyful living. It is never too late to start practising good habits and changing your life for the better. I invite you to choose one habit you didn't do, or revisit one you had trouble with and work on it. You can do it! Yes You Can.

AGE SMART FITNESS PRODUCTS

Posture, Breathing, Back Pain, Chair Program, Stretch &
Strengthen, Elastics and Weights

Age Smart Fitness Training Programs on DVD
http://www.agesmartfitness.com/store/

Age Smart Fitness Training Programs ONLINE
http://www.agesmartfitness.com/age-smart-fitness-online-classes/

www.ingramcontent.com/pod-product-compliance
Lightning Source LLC
Chambersburg PA
CBHW060902280326
41934CB00007B/1148